INTRODUCTORY CONCEPTS

IN

PATHOLOGY

INTRODUCTORY CONCEPTS

IN

PATHOLOGY

A Manual for Students
in the
Health Professions

by

LEONARD V. CROWLEY, M.D.

Attending Pathologist, St. Mary's Hospital
Clinical Assistant Professor of Laboratory Medicine,
University of Minnesota Medical School
Visiting Professor, St. Mary's Junior College, Minneapolis, Minnesota

YEAR BOOK MEDICAL PUBLISHERS · INC.

35 EAST WACKER DRIVE, CHICAGO

Library of Congress Catalog Card Number: 72-76457

International Standard Book Number: 0-8151-2031-1

Preface

THIS MANUAL is an outgrowth of a one-semester course which has been given for several years to students in nursing and other health professions at St. Mary's Junior College in Minneapolis, Minnesota. The course was designed to orient students to the fundamental concepts of disease and to provide a basic knowledge of the various types of disease which they will encounter during later contact with hospital patients. In some instances, brief comments regarding therapy have been included to illustrate how the characteristics of a disease dictate the type of treatment. The material in the manual is designed to be supplemented in class by clinical photographs, gross and microscopic photographs, and selected motion picture films, in order to provide a more graphic understanding of the effect of disease on the various organ systems.

The manual should be considered as an introduction to pathology, and not as a complete presentation of the subject. Emphasis has been placed on the more common diseases, with which the student should be familiar. Upon completion of the course, the student will have enough background to be able to expand his or her fundamental knowledge of the subject by reading any of the excellent textbooks available in pathology and in medicine. From there, he or she can gradually build upon the foundation gained in the introductory course. A selected list of reference books is included at the end of the manual as a source of more detailed information, once the student has a firm grasp of basic concepts.

I am happy to acknowledge the assistance of Sister Margaret Francis Schilling, head of the Department of Medical Photography at St. Mary's Hospital, who prepared the illustrations, and Miss Joyce Everhardt, who typed the manuscript. I would also like to thank the many students in nursing and other health fields who have made helpful suggestions, and who have assisted in designing a manual to fulfill their needs.

L. V. CROWLEY

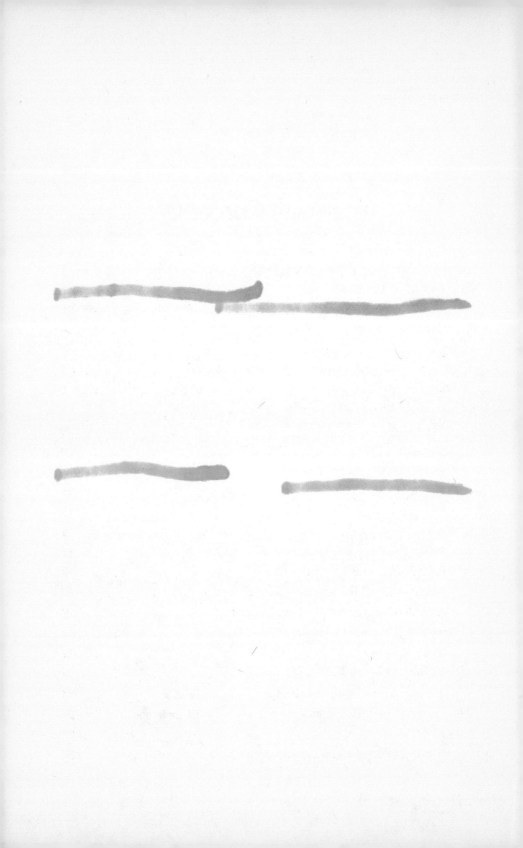

Table of Contents

Chapter 1

Introduction:

General Concepts of Disease

Characteristics of Disease

DISEASE MAY BE CONSIDERED as any disturbance of structure or function of the body. A disease is often associated with well-defined and characteristic structural changes, called *lesions,* which are present in various organs and tissues. One can recognize these by examining the diseased tissue with the naked eye or with the aid of a microscope. A disease associated with structural changes is called an *organic disease.* In contrast, a *functional disease* is one in which no morphologic abnormalities (*morphe* = structure or shape) can be identified, even though bodily functions may be profoundly disturbed. Many nervous and mental diseases are of this type. *Pathology* is the study of disease; a pathologist is a physician who specializes in the diagnosis and classification of disease, primarily by examining the morphology of cells or tissues.

A disease may cause various subjective manifestations in an affected individual, such as weakness or pain. These are called *symptoms.* A disease may also produce objective manifestations, detectable by the physician, which are called *signs* or *physical findings.* In many diseases, the numbers of blood cells in the circulation may change, as well as the biochemical constituents in the body fluids; these alterations are reflected as abnormal laboratory test results. The determination of the nature and cause of a patient's illness by a physician is called a *diagnosis.* It is based upon the physician's evaluation of the patient's subjective symptoms, the physical findings, and the results of various laboratory tests. When the physician has reached a diagnosis, he can then offer an opinion concerning the eventual outcome of the disease, which is called a *prognosis.*

Frequently, a disease causes the affected individual no discomfort nor disability. This is called an *asymptomatic* disease or illness. However, the disease may progress, if untreated, to the stage where it causes various subjective symptoms and abnormal physical findings. Therefore, the distinction between asymptomatic and symptomatic disease is one of degree, depending primarily on the extent of the disease.

The term *etiology* means cause. A disease of unknown etiology is one for which the cause is unknown. Unfortunately, many diseases fall into this category. In many diseases, the cause is known, and the agent responsible for the disease is called the *etiologic agent*. The term *pathogenesis* refers to the manner by which a disease develops.

Classification of Disease

Diseases tend to fall into several large categories. This does not imply that the diseases in a specific category are necessarily closely related. Rather, it indicates that the lesions produced by the various diseases are morphologically similar, or that the diseases have a similar pathogenesis. Diseases are conveniently classified in the following large groups: (1) congenital and hereditary diseases, (2) inflammatory diseases, (3) degenerative diseases, (4) metabolic diseases, and (5) neoplastic diseases.

CONGENITAL AND HEREDITARY DISEASES

These are the result of abnormal intrauterine development. They may result from genetic abnormalities, abnormalities in the numbers and distribution of chromosomes, or intrauterine injury due to various agents. Hemophilia, the well-known hereditary disease in which blood does not clot properly, and congenital heart disease induced by the German measles virus are examples of diseases in this category.

INFLAMMATORY DISEASES

Inflammatory diseases are those in which the body reacts to an injurious agent by means of inflammation. Many of the diseases characterized by inflammation are due to bacteria or other microbiologic agents. Others are a manifestation of an allergic reaction or a hypersensitivity state in the patient. Some diseases in this category appear to be due to antibodies formed against the patient's own tissues. The etiology of still other inflammatory diseases has not been determined.

DEGENERATIVE DISEASES

In degenerative diseases, the primary abnormality consists of degeneration of various parts of the body. In some cases, this may be a manifestation of the aging process. However, in many cases, the degenerative lesions are more advanced and occur sooner than would be expected as a result of aging, and are distinctly abnormal. Certain types of arthritis and "hardening of the arteries" are common examples of degenerative diseases.

METABOLIC DISEASES

Metabolic diseases have as their chief abnormality a disturbance in some important metabolic process in the body, such as a disturbance in the utilization of glucose by the cells or an abnormal regulation of the rate of cell metabolism by the thyroid gland. Diabetes, disturbances of endocrine glands, and disturbances of fluid and electrolyte balance are common examples of metabolic diseases.

NEOPLASTIC DISEASES

Neoplastic diseases are characterized by abnormal growth of cells, leading to the formation of various types of benign and malignant tumors.

Chapter 2

Inflammation and Repair

The Inflammatory Process

THE INFLAMMATORY REACTION is a nonspecific response to any injurious agent which causes cell death (usually called *necrosis*). The injury may be due to a physical agent (such as heat or cold), a chemical agent (such as concentrated acid or alkali or other caustic chemical), or a microbiologic agent (such as a bacterium or virus). Various substances liberated from the damaged tissue cause both local and systemic effects, as indicated diagrammatically in Figure 2-1.

Local effects consist of dilatation of capillaries and increased capillary permeability. The products of tissue necrosis also attract leukocytes to the site of injury. The characteristic signs of inflammation are heat, redness, tenderness, swelling, and pain. The increased warmth and redness of the inflamed tissues are due to dilatation of capillaries and slowing of blood flow through the vessels. The swelling is secondary to the extravasation of plasma from the dilated and more permeable capillaries, resulting in an increased volume of fluid in the inflamed tissue. The tenderness and pain are secondary to irritation of sensory nerve endings at the site of the inflammatory process.

If the inflammatory process is marked, systemic effects become evident. The individual feels ill, and the temperature is elevated. Moreover, the production of leukocytes by the bone marrow is accelerated, resulting in an increase in the number of leukocytes circulating in the blood stream.

The polymorphonuclear leukocyte is the most important cell in the acute inflammatory response. This is an actively phagocytic cell which is attracted to the area by the products of cell necrosis. Mononuclear cells (monocytes, macrophages) appear later in the inflammatory reaction and are concerned primarily with cleaning up the debris resulting from the inflammatory process. These cells are also active in chronic inflammatory reactions.

The term *infection* is used to indicate an inflammatory process due to a

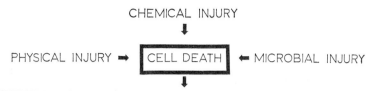

Fig. 2-1.—Local and systemic effects of cell necrosis induced by various injurious agents.

disease-producing organism. A number of different terms are used to refer to infections in various sites. Generally, the ending "itis" is appended to the name of the tissue or organ in order to indicate an infection or inflammatory process. For example, the terms appendicitis, hepatitis, colitis, and pneumonitis, refer to inflammation involving the appendix, liver, colon, and lung, respectively. An acute spreading infection in any site is called *cellulitis.* Usually this term is used when one refers to an acute infection of the skin and deeper tissues. The term *abscess* is used when an infection is associated with actual breakdown of the tissues and the formation of a localized mass of pus. If a localized infection spreads into the lymphatic channels draining the site of inflammation, the term *lymphangitis* is used. *Lymphadenitis* refers to infection in the regional lymph nodes draining the primary site of infection. The term *septicemia* is used to refer to an overwhelming infection in which pathogenic bacteria gain access to the blood stream.

In any inflammatory process, there is some degree of destruction of tissues which must be repaired. Healing consists of replacement of damaged cells and rebuilding the framework of the injured tissue by means of ingrowth of cells which produce connective tissue fibers and new blood vessels. Large areas of tissue destruction are replaced by scar tissue.

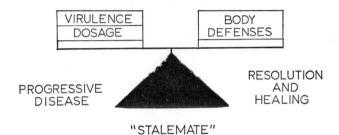

COURSE OF
INFECTION

Fig. 2-2.—Factors influencing outcome of an infection.

Factors Influencing the Outcome of an Infection

In any infection, the invading organism is pitted against the defenses of the body. Bacteria and other microbiologic agents vary in their ability to cause disease. Many are not harmful to man. Others, capable of causing disease in man, are called *pathogenic* (*pathos* = disease + *genic* = producing) organisms. The term *virulence* refers to the ease with which a pathogenic organism can overcome the defenses of the body. A highly virulent organism is one likely to produce progressive disease in most susceptible individuals. In contrast, an organism of low virulence is capable of producing disease only in a highly susceptible individual under favorable circumstances.

The outcome of any infection depends upon two factors: (1) the virulence of the organism along with the numbers ("dosage") of the invading organisms, and (2) the resistance of the infected individual (often called the *host*). These may be considered balanced against one another, as indicated diagrammatically in Figure 2-2. When large numbers of organisms of high virulence are introduced into the body, especially when host resistance is lowered, the balance is tipped in favor of the organism, and progressive or fatal disease develops. When the virulence or dosage of the organism is low, or the body's resistance is high, the balance is tipped in favor of the host. The infection is then overcome, and healing occurs.

Chronic Infection

Sometimes, the organism and host are evenly balanced against each other. Neither can gain the advantage; the result is a stalemate. Clinically, this results in a *chronic infection*, characterized by a relatively quiet, smoldering inflammation which is usually associated with vigorous attempts at healing on the part of the host. The balance between the host and invader is precarious. The infection may flare up at times when the pathogen obtains a temporary advantage, or it may become quiescent at other times when the defenses of the host gain the upper hand.

Chapter 3

Immunity and Hypersensitivity

THE BODY HAS two separate defense mechanisms for dealing with pathogenic microorganisms and other foreign, potentially harmful substances.
One mechanism consists of *phagocytosis* of the material by neutrophils
and macrophages. The second consists of the development of an *acquired
immunity*. Both mechanisms complement one another, and both function
together to protect the individual from disease.

Acquired immunity which develops after previous contact with pathogenic bacteria is only one manifestation of a person's capacity to react to
a large number of foreign antigens. Two types of acquired immunity are
recognized. One type is associated with the development of antibodies in
the serum and is called *humoral immunity*. In the second type, no antibodies are detected, but the body has developed cells which have an
enhanced ability to attack and destroy the pathogenic organisms. This is
called *cell-mediated immunity*.

Acquired immunity is often associated with a state of altered reactivity
to bacterial products or foreign material, leading to an intense inflammatory reaction at the site of contact with the foreign antigen. This increased responsiveness is called *hypersensitivity*. For example, contact
with the tubercle bacillus leads to cell-mediated immunity and is also
associated with the development of tissue hypersensitivity to antigens of
the tubercle bacillus. However, many diseases are associated with the
development of an acquired immunity without demonstrable hypersensitivity.

Immunity

THE LYMPHOCYTE AND ACQUIRED IMMUNITY

The mature lymphocyte is the most important cell concerned in the
development of acquired immunity. Two different groups of lymphocytes
are present in the body which appear identical morphologically. How-

8

ever, they are derived from different sources embryologically and have different functions. One group is concerned with the development of cell-mediated immunity. A second group develops into antibody-producing cells involved in the humoral defense reaction. Humoral and cell-mediated immunity are two basically different processes. In various diseases, either or both defense mechanisms may be impaired.

Mechanism of Production of Acquired Immunity

The initial phase in the immune defense reaction is the interaction of small lymphocytes and phagocytic reticuloendothelial cells. The phagocytic cells ingest and "process" the antigen in some manner, after which they transfer the processed antigen to the lymphocytes. The initial interaction between lymphocytes and macrophages may lead either to antibody production, cell-mediated immunity, or sometimes both types of immune defense reactions (Fig. 3-1).

Antibody Production: The Humoral Defense Reaction

After lymphocyte-macrophage interaction, the lymphocytes undergo a change in appearance (called a "transformation"), they proliferate, and they begin to produce antibody. The altered lymphocytes undergo further change into plasma cells, which also produce antibody. Once the initial phase concerned with antibody production has been completed, any subsequent contact with the antigen will lead to rapid production of antibody because the lymphoid cells have already been sensitized by previous antigenic stimulation.

Fig. 3-1.—Interrelationship of cell-mediated and humoral immunity.

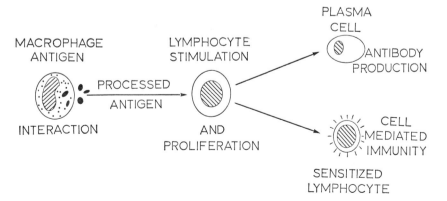

Variations in the rate of antibody production after antigenic stimulation are due to the initial lymphocyte-macrophage interaction which is followed by lymphocyte proliferation. Antigenic stimulation is succeeded by an initial lag phase of several weeks before antibodies develop, corresponding to the initial phase of lymphocyte-macrophage interaction. This is followed by a phase of rapid increase in antibody concentration, corresponding to the period of active antibody production by the proliferating lymphoid cells. Eventually a steady level of antibody production is attained, corresponding to production of antibody by plasma cells derived from the stimulated lymphocytes.

THE CELL-MEDIATED IMMUNE DEFENSE MECHANISM

After lymphocyte-macrophage interaction, the lymphocytes become sensitized and proliferate but do not differentiate into plasma cells. The stimulated lymphocytes elaborate various substances which attract and activate macrophages, causing them to function more efficiently as phagocytes against the antigenic foreign material. A similar lag phase after antigenic stimulation is seen with cell-mediated immunity, comparable to the lag associated with humoral antibody production. In cell-mediated immunity, the sensitized lymphocytes and macrophages accumulate around the antigenic foreign material. The presence of cellular immunity can be detected by the delayed hypersensitivity reaction, described below.

Cell-mediated immunity plays a major role in defenses against fungi, viruses, parasites, and mycobacteria; it is also involved in the immune defense reactions against some other bacteria. Figure 3-1 summarizes the major concepts concerning the interrelationships of cell-mediated and humoral immunity.

Hypersensitivity

Hypersensitivity is closely related to immunity. One type, immediate hypersensitivity, is associated with the presence of antibodies in the serum. Subsequent contact with the foreign protein leads to an antigen-antibody reaction causing acute respiratory distress, called *anaphylactic shock*, or a more chronic reaction characterized by hives, joint pains, and fever, called *serum sickness.*

Delayed hypersensitivity is a manifestation of cell-mediated immunity. This develops after exposure to a foreign antigen from bacteria, parasites, or other microorganisms. No antibodies are detected in the serum after sensitization, but the cells of the body have been altered as a result of exposure to the foreign protein, as described. After sensitization, subsequent contact with the antigen by injection of a test dose of antigen into the skin leads to an acute inflammatory reaction. In contrast to the immediate hypersensitivity reaction, the maximum inflammatory reaction in delayed hypersensitivity does not develop immediately, but only after 24 to 48 hours, the delay being the time necessary for the sensitized cells to accumulate at the site. This type of delayed hypersensitivity is commonly seen in tuberculosis, and is sometimes called *tuberculin-type hypersensitivity*. Hypersensitivity reactions associated with a graft of antigenically foreign tissue are of this type.

Tissue Grafts and Immunity

An individual will accept a graft of his own tissue or that of an identical twin but not that of another person. A graft from another person contains antigens foreign to the recipient. The foreign antigens cause a delayed hypersensitivity reaction characterized by infiltration of the graft by lymphoid cells and macrophages, as described. This is a manifestation of a cell-mediated immune reaction. In the treatment of patients with kidney failure, physicians can induce a patient to accept a foreign kidney, provided that his immunologic defenses have been suppressed by the administration of certain drugs or antilymphocytic serum (serum capable of destroying the host's lymphocyte defenses). The success of renal transplantation depends upon the suppression of the patient's immunologic defense mechanisms, thereby forcing him to accept antigenically foreign tissue.

Chapter 4

Autoimmune Diseases

NORMALLY, a person does not form antibodies to his own cells but only to foreign antigens, because the body has developed a tolerance to the antigens normally present within itself. However, in certain diseases the patient forms antibodies to his own cells and tissues, and the antibody injures or destroys the patient's cells or tissue components. This type of antibody is called an autoantibody (*auto* = self). Diseases associated with autoantibodies are called autoimmune diseases.

The reasons for autoantibody formation are not well understood. In some cases, certain components in the patient's own tissues appear to have been altered by disease so that they become antigenic and capable of inducing an immune response (Fig. 4-1, left). In other cases, the antibody may have been formed initially in response to a foreign antigen, but the antibody also cross-reacts with a similar antigen in the patient's own tissues, leading to tissue injury (Fig. 4-1, right).

In general, treatment of autoimmune disease is unsatisfactory. Frequently, large doses of adrenal cortical hormones are administered. These have an anti-inflammatory effect and also may suppress antibody formation. Various other drugs are sometimes administered which act by depressing the patient's ability to form antibodies.

Fig. 4-1.—Postulated mechanisms resulting in autoantibody formation.

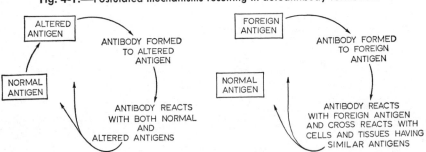

TABLE 4-1.—COMMON AUTOIMMUNE DISEASES

DISEASE	PROBABLE PATHOGENESIS	MAJOR CLINICAL MANIFESTATIONS
Rheumatic fever	Antistreptococcal antibodies cross-react with antigens in heart muscle, heart valves, and other tissues	Inflammation of heart and joints
Glomerulonephritis	Streptococci cause alteration of antigens in renal glomeruli, leading to antibody formation; antigen-antibody reaction causes glomerular injury	Inflammation of renal glomeruli
Rheumatoid arthritis	Antibodies formed against serum gamma globulin	Systemic disease with inflammation and degeneration of joints
Autoimmune blood diseases	Autoantibodies formed against platelets, white cells, or red cells; in some cases, antibody apparently was formed against altered cell antigens, and antibody reacts with both altered and normal cells	Anemia, leukopenia, or thrombocytopenia, depending on nature of antibody
Lupus erythematosus and related collagen diseases	Various antinuclear antibodies cause widespread injury to multiple organs	Systemic disease with manifestations involving multiple organs
Thyroiditis	Antithyroid antibody causes injury and inflammatory cell infiltration of thyroid gland	Hypothyroidism

Table 4-1 summarizes some of the more important diseases in which autoantibody formation appears to play a role. These diseases will be considered in greater detail in other sections of the manual.

Collagen Diseases

Collagen is the term for fibrous connective tissue which forms the framework of all tissues in the body. *Collagen disease* is a general term for a group of diseases characterized by necrosis and degeneration of collagen throughout the body. In many instances, autoantibodies directed against antigens present in various cells and tissues can be detected in the serum of affected individuals. Therefore, the collagen diseases are usually classified as autoimmune diseases.

The clinical features of the collagen disease depend upon the organ system involved and the extent of the injury to the tissues. Involvement of the connective tissue of the joints and periarticular tissues is manifested by swelling, pain, and tenderness in the joints. The cardiovascular manifestations consist of swelling and degeneration of collagen of the heart valves (leading to valve injury), inflammation of the heart muscle with degeneration of myocardial collagen, and destructive lesions involving the small and medium-sized blood vessels. Renal manifestations include inflammation and scarring of the glomeruli, damage to the glomerular basement membrane, and consequent leakage of protein and red cells into the urine. Marked glomerular damage impairs renal function and may eventually lead to renal insufficiency. Injury to the connective tissues of the lungs, pleura, and pericardium leads to pleural and pericardial pain, sometimes with accumulation of fluid in the serous cavities. Often autoantibodies directed against one or more of the formed elements in the blood may cause anemia due to increased red blood cell destruction (hemolytic anemia), reduction in platelets (thrombocytopenia), or a decrease in white cells (leukopenia).

Lupus Erythematosus

One of the more common collagen diseases is called *lupus erythematosus*. This disease is seen most frequently in young women and is characterized by widespread damage of collagen in skin, articular tissues, heart, serous membranes (pleura and pericardium), and kidney. There are frequently hematologic manifestations of anemia, leukopenia, and thrombocytopenia which are due to autoantibodies. Many patients die of renal failure resulting from the severe renal glomerular injury.

A characteristic feature of the disease is the *LE cell phenomenon*, which is due to antinucleoprotein antibodies in the patient's blood. It can be demonstrated by incubating the patient's blood serum with intact white blood cells. The antinucleoprotein antibodies damage many of the leukocytes, causing swelling and loss of structural detail in the cell nuclei. The damaged nuclei become converted into large, homogeneous, spherical "blobs" of blue-staining nuclear debris, which become surrounded and phagocytized by polymorphonuclear leukocytes. The phagocytized spherical mass fills the cytoplasm of the cell and displaces the nucleus to the edge of the cell, resulting in the characteristic appearance called an *LE cell*. A positive LE test is a valuable laboratory test for confirming the diagnosis of lupus erythematosus.

Chapter 5

Diseases Due to Bacteria

Pathogenic Organisms and Man

MAN COEXISTS with a large number of microorganisms. In most instances, man and his microbiologic associates live in harmony. Of the wide spectrum of organisms found in nature, only a relatively small proportion can cause disease in man. The pathogenic microorganisms which cause disease are classified into several large groups: viruses, rickettsiae, bacteria, and fungi. In addition, man serves as a host to a number of animal parasites capable of causing illness or disability. The various organisms which may injure man vary in their ability to cause disease. A small number of microbiologic agents are extremely virulent. Other organisms are of very low virulence and are capable of causing disease only when the body's normal defenses have been already weakened by a debilitating illness.

Classification of Bacteria

Bacteria are classified on the basis of four major characteristics: shape, gram-stain reaction, metabolic and cultural characteristics, and antigenic structure.

SHAPE

A bacterium may be spherical (coccus), rod-shaped (bacillus), or may have a spiral or corkscrew shape. Cocci may grow in clusters (staphylococci), in pairs (diplococci), or in chains (streptococci).

GRAM-STAIN REACTION

In this staining method, a dried, fixed suspension of bacteria, prepared on a microscope slide, is stained with a purple dye and then an iodine solution. Next, the slide is decolorized with alcohol or other solvent; it is then stained with a red dye. Bacteria which resist decolorization and retain the purple stain are called *gram-positive,* while those which have been decolorized and accept the red counterstain are termed *gram-negative.* By means of this staining method, all organisms may be characterized as either gram-positive or gram-negative.

BIOCHEMICAL AND CULTURAL CHARACTERISTICS

Some bacteria are quite *fastidious* and can be grown only on enriched media under carefully controlled conditions of temperature and pH. Other bacteria are hardy and capable of growing on relatively simple culture media under a wide variety of conditions.

Some bacteria are able to grow only in the absence of oxygen or under extremely low oxygen tension. These are called *anaerobic* (without oxygen) bacteria. Most bacteria grow best in the presence of oxygen (*aerobic* organisms). Others grow equally well under either aerobic or anaerobic conditions.

Many bacteria have special structural characteristics. Some form spores, spherical structures formed within the bacterial cell. Spores can survive under conditions which would kill an actively growing bacterium. They may be considered a dormant, extremely resistant form of a bacterium which forms under adverse conditions. Spores can germinate and give rise to actively growing bacteria under favorable conditions. Some bacteria have flagella; these are hair-like processes covering the surface of the bacteria. The motility of many bacteria is due to the presence of flagella. Other organisms lack flagella and are nonmotile.

Most bacteria have distinct biochemical characteristics. Various types of bacteria have the ability to ferment various carbohydrates and to bring about many different biochemical reactions when grown in suitable culture media. Each type of bacterium has its own "biochemical profile" which aids in its identification.

ANTIGENIC STRUCTURE

Each type of bacterium contains a large number of antigens associated with the cell body, the capsule of the bacterium, and the flagella (in the case of motile organisms). The antigenic structure can be determined by special methods, defining a system of antigens unique for each group of bacteria.

Identification of Bacteria

These various methods of classification can be applied to the identification of specific bacterium. Let us assume, for example, that an organism is isolated from the blood of a patient with a febrile illness. By means of the gram-stain reaction, the organism is identified as a gram-negative bacillus. The cultural characteristics indicate that it is not a fastidious organism and is capable of growing on a wide variety of culture media at various temperatures; moreover, it grows well both in the presence of oxygen or under anaerobic conditions. The organism is motile and does not form spores.

At this point, the number of possible organisms consistent with these characteristics has been reduced to relatively few gram-negative bacteria. The number of possibilities is narrowed still further by the performance of various biochemical tests which indicate that the bacterium does not ferment lactose but is able to ferment glucose and certain other sugars. These and other biochemical tests permit the conclusion that the organism is a type of pathogenic bacterium called *Salmonella*, found in the gastrointestinal tract and capable of causing a typhoid-like, febrile illness. The various bacterial antigens within the cell body and flagella of the bacteria can be identified; these allow a determination of the exact type of *Salmonella* responsible for the patient's illness.

Once the organism has been identified, the physician can begin proper treatment and can institute proper isolation and control procedures, based on a knowledge of how the disease is transmitted.

Diseases Caused by Pathogenic Bacteria

The following is a summary of the diseases which are caused by the more important bacteria which infect man. A brief classification of the major pathogenic bacteria is indicated in Table 5-1.

TABLE 5-1.—IMPORTANT PATHOGENIC BACTERIA

TYPE	GRAM-STAIN REACTION	
	Gram-Positive	Gram-Negative
Cocci	Staphylococci	Gonococci
	Streptococci	Meningococci
	Pneumococci	
Bacilli	Diphtheria bacillus (aerobic)	Small fastidious bacteria
		Hemophilus
	Clostridia (anaerobic)	*Pasteurella*
		Brucella
		Enteric bacteria
		Salmonella-Shigella-Cholera bacillus
		Colon bacillus and related organisms
Spiral Organisms	*Treponema pallidum*	
Acid-fast organisms	Tubercle bacillus	
	Leprosy bacillus	

STAPHYLOCOCCI

Staphylococci are the normal inhabitants of the skin and nasal cavity. They are a common cause of boils, various other skin infections, and postoperative wound infections. Occasionally, staphylococci cause serious pulmonary infections and other types of systemic infections. Staphylococcal infections often pose a serious problem in hospitals because the organisms are widely distributed and many hospitalized patients are unusually susceptible to infection. Many patients have had recent surgical operations; others have various chronic diseases associated with impairment of the body's normal defenses against bacterial infection. Some strains of staphylococci are highly resistant to antibiotics, and infections due to antibiotic-resistant staphylococci are extremely difficult to treat.

STREPTOCOCCI

There are many kinds of streptococci which vary in their pathogenicity. These organisms are subdivided into a large number of serologic types on the basis of their antigenic structure. They are also classified on the basis of their cultural characteristics when grown on a solid media containing blood. *Alpha hemolytic streptococci* produce green discoloration of the blood immediately around the colony. These organisms are normal inhabitants of the upper respiratory tract and are not normally pathogenic. *Beta hemolytic streptococci* produce a narrow zone of complete hemolysis of blood around the growing colony. Many strains of beta streptococci are extremely pathogenic, causing streptococcal sore throat, scarlet fever, serious skin infections, and infections of the uterus after childbirth. Some strains of beta streptococci are capable of inducing a state of hypersensitivity in susceptible individuals, leading to the development of rheumatic fever or a type of kidney disease called glomerulonephritis. These diseases will be considered in greater detail in the sections on the circulatory system (Chapter 15) and kidney (Chapter 22). *Gamma streptococci* cause no changes in the blood medium surrounding the bacterial colony; thus, they are often referred to as *nonhemolytic streptococci*. In general, these organisms are nonpathogenic.

PNEUMOCOCCI

Pneumococci are gram-positive cocci which grow in pairs and short chains and have certain biochemical characteristics setting them apart from streptococci. Pneumococci are a common cause of bacterial pneumonia.

GRAM-NEGATIVE COCCI

Most gram-negative cocci are nonpathogenic members of the genus *Neisseria* and are normal inhabitants of the upper respiratory passages. This group contains two pathogenic members. The meningococcus (*Neisseria meningiditis*) causes a type of meningitis (inflammation of the membranes surrounding the brain and spinal cord), frequently occurring in epidemics. The gonococcus (*Neisseria gonorrhoeae*) causes gonorrhea. This disease is transmitted by sexual contact and will be discussed in greater detail in the sections on the reproductive system (Chapters 20 and 23).

GRAM-POSITIVE BACILLI

AEROBIC NON-SPORE-FORMING GRAM-POSITIVE BACILLI.—Members of this group are called *corynebacteria*. Most are nonpathogenic inhabitants of the upper respiratory passages. However, one member of the group (*Corynebacterium diphtheriae*) causes diphtheria. This organism causes an acute ulcerative inflammation of the throat and also produces a potent toxin which can injure heart muscle and nerve tissue.

ANAEROBIC SPORE-FORMING GRAM-POSITIVE BACILLI.—Anaerobic spore-forming bacilli are called *clostridia*. These are normal inhabitants of the intestinal tract of man and animals and are also found in the soil. Members of this group produce potent toxins and cause several important diseases. Some bacteria in this group cause gas gangrene, some cause tetanus (lockjaw), and others cause botulism.

Gas gangrene.—Gas gangrene develops in dirty wounds contaminated with certain species of clostridia. These anaerobic organisms grow in dead or devitalized tissue, especially in wounds where considerable necrosis of muscle has taken place. The clostridia produce large amounts of gas from fermentation of the necrotic tissues and also liberate powerful toxins with widespread systemic effects.

Tetanus.—One species of clostridia produces a potent toxin which causes spasm of voluntary muscles. The common term *lockjaw* comes from the marked rigidity of the jaw muscles, a common feature of this disease. Tetanus may be fatal because of respiratory failure resulting from spasm of the muscles concerned with respiration.

Botulism.—The *Clostridium botulinum* produces a potent neuroparalytic toxin. Generally botulism can be traced to eating improperly processed or canned foods in which the organism has grown and produced toxin. Botulism is actually a poisoning due to the ingestion of toxin in food, rather than a bacterial infection. Recently, outbreaks of botulism have been traced to contamination of canned tuna fish and canned soup prepared in commercial canneries.

GRAM-NEGATIVE BACTERIA

FASTIDIOUS ORGANISMS.—Three separate groups of small fastidious gram-negative bacteria are of clinical importance. These are named *Hemophilus, Pasteurella,* and *Brucella.* Members of the genus *Hemophilus* are normal inhabitants of the respiratory tract. One member of this group, *Hemophilus influenzae,* sometimes causes meningitis in infants and young children. Occasionally, it produces respiratory infections in patients with chronic lung disease. One member of the genus *Pasteurella* is responsible for bubonic plague. Another member of the genus produces a somewhat similar illness called tularemia. Members of the genus *Brucella* cause disease in animals which can be transmitted to man. The disease in man, undulant fever, is a febrile illness; it is contracted from drinking unpasteurized milk obtained from infected animals.

THE ENTERIC BACTERIA.—The enteric bacteria constitute a number of closely related organisms distinguishable by their biochemical and serologic characteristics. Many of these organisms are inhabitants of the gastrointestinal tract of man and animals. Other members of the group are free-living organisms, widely distributed in nature. Three members of this group, *Salmonella, Shigella,* and the cholera bacillus (*Vibrio comma*), are pathogenic, causing various types of febrile illness and gastroenteritis. The organisms are excreted from the gastrointestinal tract in the feces of infected patients; transmission occurs by means of food or water contaminated by the organisms.

Other members of this large group are of only limited pathogenicity, but sometimes produce disease when they are outside of their normal habitat in the gastrointestinal tract. These organisms may cause wound infections, urinary tract infections, and pulmonary infections in susceptible individuals. The best-known member of this group is the colon bacillus, which is the predominant organism found within the intestinal tract of man and animals.

SPIRAL ORGANISMS

The spiral organisms can cause a wide variety of illnesses. The best-known member of this group is *Treponema pallidum,* which causes syphilis. The disease is spread by sexual contact, the organism being introduced through a break in the mucous membrane of the genital tract. After an incubation period of several weeks, a localized area of inflammation (called a chancre) containing large numbers of organisms develops at the site of the inoculation. After several more weeks, the infected person develops symptoms of a systemic infection due to widespread dissemination of the organisms throughout the body. The disease at this stage is highly infectious and is characterized by enlarged lymph nodes, fever, and various types of skin rashes. Eventually, after many years, if the disease is not treated, late destructive lesions may develop involving the nervous system and the cardiovascular system.

A syphilitic mother may transmit the disease to her unborn infant. This may cause intrauterine fetal death, or the infant may be born alive with congenital syphilis.

ACID-FAST BACTERIA

The best-known acid-fast bacterium is the tubercle bacillus, responsible for tuberculosis. Certain other organisms in this group also produce a tuberculosis-like disease in man. Another acid-fast bacterium causes leprosy.

These organisms have a waxy capsule which is stained with difficulty by means of certain red dyes. Once the organism has been stained, the stain-impregnated capsule resists decolorization with various acid solvents. This property, attributable to the capsule, is responsible for the term *acid-fast* used to refer to this type of organism. Acid-fast bacteria cause a special type of chronic inflammatory reaction, called a chronic granulomatous inflammation, rather than the usual polymorphonuclear inflammatory reaction seen with most bacterial infections.

Chapter 6

Treatment of Bacterial Infections with Antibiotics

THE DISCOVERY OF antibiotic compounds and their widespread use in the treatment of various types of infections has been one of the great advances in medicine. Antibiotics are substances which destroy bacteria or inhibit bacterial growth. They are useful clinically because of their ability to injure bacterial cells without producing significant injury to the patient.

Mode of Action

The bacterial cell is a complex structure containing genetic material, a protein-synthesizing mechanism, numerous enzyme systems concerned with various intracellular metabolic functions, a semipermeable cell membrane, and a rigid cell wall. Antimicrobial substances act by interfering with the structure or function of the bacterial cell by one or more of the following methods (Fig. 6-1):

Fig. 6-1.—Various sites of action of antibiotics, as described in text. Antibiotics may act by disrupting the bacterial cell wall, by disturbing the functions of the cell membrane, or by interfering with the intracellular "metabolic machinery." Some antimicrobial drugs are not directly injurious to the bacterial cell, but compete with essential substances required for bacterial growth and multiplication.

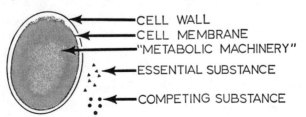

CELL WALL
CELL MEMBRANE
"METABOLIC MACHINERY"
ESSENTIAL SUBSTANCE
COMPETING SUBSTANCE

INHIBITION OF CELL-WALL SYNTHESIS

The bacterial cell has a high internal osmotic pressure, and the rigid outer cell wall maintains the shape of the bacterium. In some respects, the function of the cell wall can be compared to a corset or girdle, supporting the enclosed cell. Penicillin and several other antibiotics act by inhibiting the synthesis of the bacterial cell wall, which exposes the bacterial cell body. Because of the high osmotic pressure of the bacterium, the relatively unsupported cell swells and eventually ruptures.

INHIBITION OF CELL-MEMBRANE FUNCTION

The cell membrane is a semipermeable membrane surrounding the bacterial protoplasm. It controls the internal composition of the cell by regulating the diffusion of materials in and out of the cell. Some antibiotics act by inhibiting various functions of the cell membrane. Loss of the selective permeability of the cell membrane leads to cell injury and death.

INHIBITION OF METABOLIC FUNCTIONS OF THE BACTERIUM

Some antibiotics interfere with nucleic acid or protein synthesis by bacteria so that the organisms are unable to carry out essential metabolic functions.

COMPETITIVE INHIBITION

Some antibiotics resemble important compounds required by bacteria for growth and multiplication. The bacteria are unable to distinguish between the essential compound and the antibiotic which resembles it, but the antibiotic cannot be substituted for the required compound in the metabolic process. When the bacteria use the "wrong" compound rather than the "correct" substance, bacterial metabolism is disrupted, leading to inhibition of bacterial growth.

Bacterial Resistance

Some bacteria which are initially sensitive to antibiotics eventually become resistant. An adaptation occurs by which the bacteria develop methods for circumventing the effect of an antibiotic. This may be due to the development of an enzyme system which inactivates the antibiotic. For example, a bacterium which was penicillin-sensitive may develop an enzyme penicillinase which inactivates the antibiotic and allows the bacteria to survive in the presence of the drug. Another method by which

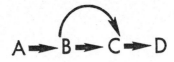

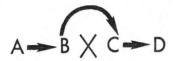

Fig. 6-2.—One method by which bacteria become resistant to antibiotics. **Above,** a bacterium carries out essential metabolic functions by means of a series of biochemical reactions. In this example, the intermediate step B $\rightarrow$ C can proceed by two alternate routes, but normally the "direct" route is favored. **Below,** if the "direct" route is blocked by the action of an antibiotic, the alternate metabolic pathway is utilized. Eventually the bacterium is able to resume its metabolic processes by "detouring around" the site of the block.

bacteria become resistant is by developing an alternate metabolic pathway for carrying out an essential function that has been blocked by an antibiotic. For example, if an antibiotic blocks a single step in a complex sequence, the bacterium may develop a metabolic pathway which detours around the site of block, allowing the metabolic process to continue by the alternate route (Fig. 6-2).

Adverse Effects of Antibiotics

Toxicity

Antibiotics are useful because they are much more toxic to bacteria than they are to the patient. Antibiotics vary in their effects upon humans, but all have some degree of toxicity. Some injure the kidneys; others injure nerve tissue or the blood-forming tissues. Penicillin and other antibiotics which act by interfering with bacterial cell wall synthesis are relatively nontoxic, probably because the animal cell has no structure comparable to the bacterial cell wall. Some antibiotics which interfere with bacterial metabolic functions can at times produce similar derangements in the patient's own metabolic functions. For example, tetracycline is a relatively nontoxic antibiotic, excreted chiefly by the kidneys. If renal function is impaired, very high blood levels of antibiotic may develop after administration of the usual therapeutic doses of the drug; this may cause severe and often fatal impairment of the patient's own cellular metabolic functions.

HYPERSENSITIVITY

Some antibiotics induce a marked hypersensitivity. This can lead to a fatal reaction if the drug is later administered to a sensitized patient. Penicillin is capable of inducing extremely severe anaphylactic reactions, although the antibiotic itself has a very low toxicity.

ALTERATION OF NORMAL BACTERIAL FLORA

The normal bacterial flora in the oral cavity, colon, and other locations may be altered by antibiotics. If the normal bacteria are destroyed, there may be overgrowth of resistant bacteria and fungi previously controlled by the normal flora. These resistant organisms may cause infections in susceptible patients.

DEVELOPMENT OF RESISTANT STRAINS OF BACTERIA

Widespread use of an antibiotic predisposes to the development of resistant strains, by mechanisms discussed previously. This may complicate the treatment of patients who become infected with antibiotic-resistant organisms. Staphylococci, in particular, have raised this problem, since many strains isolated from hospital patients are highly resistant to a large number of antibiotics. Treatment of gonorrhea has also been complicated by the development of a high degree of penicillin resistance in many strains of gonococci, so that prolonged courses of therapy and much larger doses of antibiotic are required to eradicate the infections. Resistant strains of tubercle bacilli have also developed, hindering the treatment of tuberculosis with antituberculous drugs. On the other hand, many bacteria have demonstrated no tendency to develop resistance to antibiotics. For example, beta streptococci remain quite sensitive to penicillin, despite widespread use of penicillin to treat streptococcal infections. *Treponema pallidum*, the organism responsible for syphilis, has also remained quite sensitive to penicillin, even though this drug has been used to treat syphilis for many years.

Indications for Antibiotic Use

Antibiotics are used by the physician to treat infections caused by susceptible bacteria. The physician is aided in his choice of the proper antibiotic by means of antibiotic sensitivity tests. In these tests, the bacteria are grown in the laboratory and tested against a number of antibiotics. A bacterium is considered sensitive to an antibiotic if bacterial growth is inhibited in the presence of the antibiotic, whereas a resistant organism will grow in the presence of the drug.

Because of the problems of toxicity from antibiotics, possible hypersensitivity reactions, problems related to overgrowth of bacterial flora, and development of resistant strains, these life-saving drugs should not be used indiscriminately. They should be administered only when there is a recognized indication.

Chapter 7

Fungus Infections

FUNGI ARE CLASSIFIED as plants without chlorophyll and are widely distributed in nature. Some fungi, such as those causing athlete's foot, live on the skin and only occasionally cause minor discomfort. Others are found in small numbers in the oral cavity, gastrointestinal tract, and vagina, where they live together in harmony with the normal bacterial flora. Most fungi have a limited ability to cause disease. However, under special circumstances, fungi may produce serious localized or systemic infection in susceptible individuals. Two major factors are known to predispose to systemic fungus infection: (1) disturbance in the normal bacterial flora, and (2) impaired immunologic defenses.

After intensive therapy with broad-spectrum antibiotics, the normal bacterial flora of the oral cavity, colon, vagina, and other areas may be altered or completely eradicated, disturbing the normal balance between the bacterial flora and fungi. Normally, the predominance of the bacterial flora hold the fungi in check. When the bacteria are eliminated, the fungi may proliferate and cause disease.

Patients with various types of chronic debilitating diseases may be susceptible to fungus infections. Infections of this type are also encountered in patients whose immunologic defense mechanisms have been depressed by various drugs, chemicals, or radiation therapy. Patients with certain types of cancer, particularly those treated with various toxic drugs, may also develop systemic fungus infections.

Highly Pathogenic Fungi

Although most fungi are at best only potential pathogens of low virulence, two are highly infectious and frequently produce disease in man. The fungus *Histoplasma capsulatum* is found in many parts of the country and causes the disease *histoplasmosis*. This organism is found in the soil and in the excreta from birds and other animals. Man becomes in-

27

fected by inhaling dust containing dried spores of the fungus. In most cases the fungus produces an acute, self-limited respiratory infection. Occasionally, progressive, disseminated, sometimes fatal disease develops. Another fungus, *Coccidioides immitis*, which is found in parts of California and elsewhere in the southwestern portion of the United States, causes the disease *coccidioidomycosis*. As in the case of histoplasmosis, man becomes infected by inhaling dust containing dried spores. The disease is similar to histoplasmosis, usually manifested as an acute pulmonary infection. However, the fungus sometimes causes severe progressive systemic disease.

Chapter 8

Viral and Rickettsial Diseases

Viruses

THE NATURE OF VIRUSES

VIRUSES ARE the smallest infectious agents, being composed of a central core consisting of nucleic acid (the genome) covered by a protein shell (the capsid). The capsid, which is discarded when the virus invades the cell, covers the virus nucleic acid, permitting survival of the virus outside of the cell. Viruses vary greatly in size. The smallest are only slightly larger than protein molecules, while the largest viruses approach the size of bacteria. Viruses have no metabolic enzymes and therefore are unable to carry out metabolic processes. The viral nucleic acid causes the normal metabolic processes of the invaded cell to be diverted to producing more viral nucleic acids and also induces the formation of virus capsular protein. The number of new proteins synthesized by the infected cell depends upon the size and complexity of the viral genome. In some instances, the virus has been shown to actually be incorporated into the nucleoprotein genetic structure of the cell. In many respects, the virus may be likened to a criminal who takes over a business, forcing it to function for his benefit rather than for the benefit of the owners.

MODE OF ACTION OF VIRUSES

A distinction is commonly made between a virus infection and a virus disease. A virus may infect a cell without causing any evidence of cell injury; this is considered a latent virus infection. Apparently, many viruses are capable of coexisting with normal cells in lymphoid tissue, the gastrointestinal tract, and probably other sites without causing cellular injury. Other types of virus are more virulent and regularly produce cell injury, manifested by necrosis and degeneration of the infected cell (called a *cytopathogenic effect*). Other viruses induce cell hyperplasia and proliferation rather than cell necrosis. Many viruses induce various combinations of cell damage and cell hyperplasia.

Under certain circumstances, a latent asymptomatic virus infection may become activated, leading to actual disease. For example, the herpes virus, which causes fever blisters, may persist in the tissues of the host for many years. The virus periodically becomes activated during an intercurrent febrile illness or when the patient's immunological defenses have been disrupted by neoplasm or by various other diseases.

INCLUSION BODIES IN VIRUS DISEASE

Tissues which are infected with virus frequently contain spherical, densely staining structures called *inclusion bodies*. These are present within the nucleus, the cytoplasm, or in both locations within the infected cell. They represent masses of virus or products of virus multiplication. The presence of inclusion bodies may be of considerable diagnostic aid in recognizing virus infection and determining the types of virus disease present.

RECOVERY FROM VIRUS INFECTION

Recovery from virus infection is associated with a production of a protein (interferon) by infected cells. Apparently this material prevents viral multiplication and eventually leads to decline of virus in tissues and recovery from infection. Adrenal cortical steroids inhibit interferon synthesis, perhaps explaining the adverse effect of cortical steroids on virus infection in man. Many virus infections are associated with an immunity to reinfection. In some cases, this may be due to persistence of the virus in the host.

UNUSUAL MANIFESTATIONS OF VIRUS INFECTION

Certain viruses are known to cause tumors in animals. It appears likely that at least some tumors in humans may also prove to be due to viruses. Moreover, some viruses have been found recently to produce very slowly progressive lesions which may require many years to develop. These are termed *slow-virus infections*. Certain types of neurologic diseases in animals are due to infections of this type, and evidence exists that some progressive neurologic diseases in humans may also be due to the action of slow viruses.

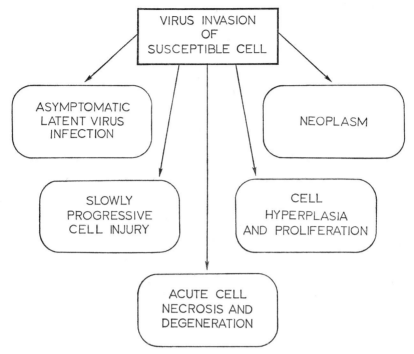

Fig. 8-1.—Summary of possible effects of a virus infection on susceptible cells.

Classification of Viruses

An older classification of viruses was based on the major clinical features of the virus infection, and viruses were classified on the basis of the portion of the body or organ system in which the virus infection produced the most prominent clinical manifestations. In this classification, viruses were classified as *dermatropic, neurotropic, pneumotropic,* or *viscerotropic.* Dermatropic infections were manifested primarily by skin rashes, such as smallpox, chickenpox, and measles. Neurotropic infections involved primarily nerve tissue, examples being rabies, poliomyelitis, and viral encephalitis. Pneumotropic infections affected primarily the respiratory system, producing the common cold, influenza, virus pneumonia, *etc.* Viscerotropic infections involved a major organ in the body, for example, the liver (hepatitis), or salivary glands (mumps).

A more modern classification categorizes viruses on the basis of their nucleic acid structure, size, structural configuration, and biologic characteristics. In this classification, several large groups of viruses are recognized, and a large number of viruses are identified in each group.

Rickettsiae

The rickettsiae are very small, intracellular parasites. Although they are usually discussed along with the viruses, they are much more closely related to bacteria. They are parasites of insects and are transmitted to man by insect bites. The organisms multiply in the endothelial cells of small blood vessels which become swollen and necrotic, leading to thrombosis, rupture, and necrosis. Clinically, a rickettsial infection usually causes a febrile illness, often associated with a skin rash. Typhus and Rocky Mountain spotted fever are the most common rickettsial diseases.

Chapter 9

Animal Parasites

ANIMAL PARASITES are organisms which have become adapted to living within the body of another animal, called the host. These organisms are no longer capable of free-living existence. Many animal parasites have a complex life cycle. Immature forms of the parasite may spend a portion of their cycle within the body of an animal or fish (the intermediate host) before the mature parasite eventually takes up residence within the body of the final host (the definitive host). In general, many animal parasites live within the intestinal tract and discharge eggs in the feces. Transmission is favored by conditions of poor sanitation and also by relatively high temperature and humidity, which enhances survival of the parasite in its infective stage. Therefore, many parasitic infestations are common in tropical climates, but are much less frequent in cold or temperate climates.

Animal parasites may be classified into two large groups: (1) the *protozoa*, which are simple, one-cell organisms, and (2) the *metazoa*, which are more complex, multicelled structures.

Protozoal Infestations

The two most important protozoal infestations in man are malaria, caused by various species of *Plasmodium*, and amebic dysentery, caused by a pathogenic ameba, *Entamoeba histolytica*.

MALARIA

Malaria, caused by several species of the protozoan parasite *Plasmodium*, is transmitted from man to man by the bite of a mosquito and parasitizes the red cells of the host, causing destruction of the red cells and an acute febrile illness. Sometimes malaria is transmitted by blood transfusions if the blood donor carries the malaria parasite. Recently, malarial infections have been encountered in drug addicts and have been traced

33

to the use of a common hypodermic syringe by several addicts, the parasite having been transferred from a carrier of the parasite to other addicts by means of the contaminated syringe.

AMEBIASIS

Amebiasis is an infection of the intestinal tract by a pathogenic ameba, *Entamoeba histolytica*. The parasite exists in an active, motile, vegetative phase (called a trophozoite) and a relatively resistant cystic phase. Man becomes infected by the ingestion of cysts of the parasite in contaminated food and water. The motile phase of the parasite develops from the cyst and invades the mucosa of the colon, producing mucosal ulcers and causing symptoms of inflammation of the colon. Occasionally, the amebas are carried to the liver in the portal circulation and may cause amebic hepatitis or amebic liver abscess.

Metazoal Infestations

The three large groups of metazoal parasites are the roundworms, the tapeworms, and the flukes.

ROUNDWORMS

The three most important roundworms which parasitize man are the *Ascaris*, the pinworm, and the *Trichinella* worm.

ASCARIS.—The *Ascaris* is a large roundworm, about the size of an earthworm, which lives within the intestinal tract and discharges eggs in the feces. Man becomes infected by the ingestion of material contaminated with *Ascaris* eggs. The worms hatch within the intestinal tract, and the small larval worms burrow through the intestine, enter the circulatory system and are carried in the circulation throughout the body. They are then filtered out in various organs and tissues. The larvae which lodge in the lung migrate into the bronchi, are coughed up, and eventually are swallowed, finding their way again into the intestinal tract where they grow to maturity. The stage characterized by the passage of immature *Ascaris* larvae through the lungs and other tissues of the host is called the phase of larval migration and is associated with fever, increase in eosinophils in the blood, and severe systemic symptoms.

Dogs and cats may be infested with a similar type of roundworm; the animal worm occasionally causes disease in humans. Infestation by the animal worm is most common in children who are in close contact with an infected animal. The children transfer the eggs to their mouth by means of contaminated hands, toys, or other objects. The eggs hatch within the intestinal tract, and the larvae invade the tissues of the host, undergoing a phase of larval migration, which is associated with severe systemic symptoms. However, the larvae which have been ingested by a foreign host are eventually destroyed within the tissues of the host and never reach maturity within the intestinal tract.

PINWORMS.—Infestation by the small roundworm, the pinworm, is frequent in children, and spread of infestation is common among members of a family. The worm measures less than 1 cm in length and lives in the colon. The parasite frequently migrates out of the colon through the anus, while the infected individual is asleep, and deposits its eggs on the perianal skin. Sometimes the worm migrates into the vagina, through the fallopian tubes, and into the peritoneal cavity, but this is uncommon. The main symptoms of pinworm infestation are intense anal and perianal itching due to irritation resulting from the migration of the worm. A person becomes infected with the worm by ingestion of eggs which are transferred to the hands from contaminated bed clothing or other objects. The disease is more of a nuisance than a threat to life.

TRICHINELLA.—Another small roundworm, the *Trichinella spiralis*, causes a severe parasitic infestation (trichinosis). The organism parasitizes not only man, but also a large number of animals. *Trichinella* are present as small cystic structures within muscles of the host. Man usually becomes infected from eating improperly cooked pork. After ingestion of the infected meat, the cysts develop into parasitic worms in the intestinal tract. The worms penetrate the intestinal wall, gain access to the circulation, are carried throughout the body, and lodge in various tissues where they incite an intense inflammatory reaction. The parasites eventually undergo cyst formation in the muscles of the infected individual. The phase of migration of the parasite is associated with severe systemic symptoms, and there may also be symptoms referable to disturbed function of organs which have been heavily infiltrated with parasites. Extremely heavy parasitic infestations may be fatal.

TAPEWORMS

Tapeworms are long, ribbon-like worms, sometimes growing to a length of several feet, which inhabit the intestinal tract of man. In general, tapeworms cause no great inconvenience to the individual carrying the worm except for depriving the host of nutrition which is used to nourish the worm. Three species of tapeworms are recognized: the pork tapeworm, the beef tapeworm, and the fish tapeworm. Man becomes infected by eating the flesh of the infected animal which contains the larval form of the parasite.

FLUKES

Flukes are large, fleshy, short worms which are provided with suckers for the attachment to the host. They have a complex life cycle involving one or more intermediate hosts. Flukes are classified according to the area of the body in which the development of the adult flukes is completed and their eggs are deposited. Some species of flukes live within the intestinal tract; others live within the liver; one species lives within the lung. Some flukes live within the portal venous system and its tributaries. Fluke infestations are important causes of disability and illness in some Asiatic countries, but human fluke infestations are not seen in this part of the world

Chapter 10

Communicable Disease

AN INFECTIOUS DISEASE which is readily transmitted from person to person is considered a communicable disease. Such a disease is said to be endemic (*en* = within + *demos* = population) if small numbers of cases are present continually in the population. It reaches epidemic proportions (*epi* = upon + *demos* = population) when relatively large numbers of people are affected. Sometimes an endemic disease may flare up and assume epidemic proportions.

Methods of Transmission

A communicable disease may be transmitted from person to person by either direct or indirect methods. Direct transmission occurs either by direct physical contact or by means of droplet spread, as by coughing or

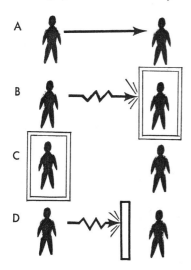

Fig. 10-1.—Various methods used to eradicate or control a communicable disease, as described in text. **A,** unimpeded direct or indirect transmission of a communicable disease from person to person. **B,** immunization protects susceptible person by conferring resistance to infection. **C,** isolation and prompt treatment of infected individual prevents spread of disease to susceptible persons. **D,** control of means of indirect transmission blocks spread of the infectious agent.

sneezing. Indirect transmission of an infectious agent is accomplished by some intermediary mechanism, such as transmission in contaminated water or by means of insects. A few communicable diseases are primarily diseases of animals and are transmitted to man only incidentally.

For a communicable disease to perpetuate itself, there must be a continuous transmission of the infectious agent from person to person by either direct or indirect methods. Therefore, in order to eradicate or control the disease, the chain of transmission must be broken at some point (Fig. 10-1).

Methods of Control

The following are some of the methods which can be applied to the control of a communicable disease. In practice, multiple methods of control are applied whenever possible.

IMMUNIZATION

If a large proportion of the population can be immunized against a communicable disease, the disease will eventually die out, since there will be very few susceptible persons in the population. Smallpox and poliomyelitis are examples of diseases that have been almost completely eradicated in this country as a result of widespread immunization.

Immunization can also be used to protect susceptible persons entering a foreign country where a communicable disease is endemic. The immunized person will no longer be susceptible to the disease, even though the disease is widespread in the native population.

IDENTIFICATION, ISOLATION, AND TREATMENT OF INFECTED PERSONS

The sick person is identified and treated promptly in order to shorten the time during which he can infect others. Isolation of the infected person prevents contact with susceptible persons and stops the spread of the disease. These are the primary methods used to control diseases when effective methods of immunization are not available. In some cases, these measures are difficult to accomplish, since some diseases produce relatively few symptoms in the infected individual. For example, the person infected with tuberculosis or a venereal disease may spread the disease to others but his own disease may not be recognized and treated because he does not feel ill and does not seek medical treatment.

CONTROL OF MEANS OF INDIRECT TRANSMISSION OF DISEASE

Various control measures can be instituted, depending upon the manner by which the infectious agent is transmitted. Where the transmission occurs via contaminated food or water, methods of control involve chlorination of water supplies and establishing effective sewage treatment facilities, control of food handlers, and standards for controlling the manufacture and distribution of commercially prepared foods. When a disease is transmitted by insects, either from man to man or from infected animals to man, it is necessary to eradicate or control the insects which transmit the disease. When a disease is spread from animals to man, control of the animal source of infection is also required.

REQUIREMENTS FOR EFFECTIVE CONTROL OF A COMMUNICABLE DISEASE

Application of effective control measures requires a knowledge of the cause of the disease and its method of transmission. If this information is not available, control measures are often ineffective. For example, bubonic plague, the "black death" of the Middle Ages, decimated entire populations because the people understood neither the cause of the disease nor how it was transmitted and therefore were unable to protect themselves from its ravages. We now know that plague is primarily a disease of rats and other rodents, that it is caused by a bacterium, and that it is transmitted to man by insects. In some cases, the plague bacillus causes a pulmonary infection in man. When this occurs, direct transmission from man to man is possible by droplet spread, causing an extremely contagious and highly fatal pulmonary infection called pneumonic plague. In some parts of the country, plague infection still persists in some rodent populations, but plague is no longer a serious problem because the disease in man can be largely prevented by control of the infected animal population and by instituting measures which prevent close contact between potentially infected rodents and man. Transmission from man to man is prevented by prompt isolation and treatment of infected persons.

Chapter 11

Congenital and Hereditary Diseases

Chromosomes

CELL DIVISION

THE STRUCTURE, differentiation, and activities of the cell are controlled by chromosomes present in the nucleus of the cell. In the somatic cell, chromosomes exist in pairs, one member of each pair having been derived from the male parent and one member from the female parent. Each member of the pair is similar in size, shape, and appearance except in the case of the sex chromosomes. In the human, the normal chromosome composition is 22 pairs of *autosomes* (a general term for chromosomes other than the sex chromosomes) and one pair of sex chromosomes.

The chromosomes are composed of double coils of deoxyribonucleic acid (DNA). In the resting, nondividing cell they are long and thin, and the individual chromosomes cannot be visualized. Genes are conceived of as arranged along the chromosome like beads on a string.

There are two types of cell division. *Mitosis,* the type of cell division characteristic of somatic cells, is cell division in which the chromosomes divide and each daughter cell receives the same number of chromosomes as the parent cell. *Meiosis* is a specialized type of cell division characteristic of germinal tissue in which the number of chromosomes is reduced so that the daughter cell receives half the chromosome content of the parent cell. Meiosis not only serves the need for reducing the chromosome number of the germ cell, it also provides for an interchange of genetic material at random between homologous chromosomes. This vastly increases the possibilities for genetic variation. Each germ cell receives at random one or the other homologous chromosome; these homologues may themselves have already been altered through reciprocal exchange of segments.

SEX DETERMINATION

Genetic sex is determined by the composition of the X and Y chromosomes. The individual having two X chromosomes is genetically female; the male has one X and one Y chromosome. After a very early stage of fetal development, only one X chromosome is necessary for normal female sexual development. The other X chromosome becomes inactive and appears as a condensation of chromatin on the nuclear membrane of the somatic cells. This condensation of chromatin is referred to as a *sex chromatin body* or *Barr body*. It is possible to determine the sex of an individual from an examination of his cells for the presence of the sex chromatin body. This is most conveniently accomplished by examining cells obtained by scraping gently the mucosa of the mouth with a tongue depressor and preparing slides from this material. However, cells obtained from any convenient site may be used for examination.

ABNORMALITIES OF CHROMOSOME DISTRIBUTION

Occasionally homologous chromosomes in germinal cells fail to separate from one another in either the first or second meiotic division. This results in abnormalities in the distribution of chromosomes between germ cells. One of the two germ cells derived from the abnormal chromosome division will have an extra chromosome, and the other cell will be lacking a chromosome. Failure of chromosome separation is called *nondisjunction* and may involve either the sex chromosomes or the autosomes. Individuals with an abnormal sex chromosome composition have been recognized. They have characteristic abnormalities of body form and usually show evidence of abnormal sexual development. Two of the more common types of sex chromosome abnormalities are the presence of an extra X chromosome in a male (sex chromosome pattern XXY, called Klinefelter's syndrome) and absence of one X chromosome in a female (sex chromosome pattern XO, called Turner's syndrome).

Mongolism is a clinical syndrome characterized by mental retardation, a characteristic facial appearance, and often various other congenital abnormalities. In most cases, mongolism (also called Down's syndrome) is due to autosomal nondisjunction, leading to an extra 21st chromosome. The affected individual has 47 rather than the normal 46 chromosomes. The presence of an extra chromosome is called a *trisomy* (*tri* = three + *soma* = body); therefore, the syndrome is also called *trisomy 21*.

In some patients with mongolism, the extra chromosome is found attached to one of the other chromosomes. In these subjects, although the total number of chromosomes is not increased, one chromosome is represented by the fusion of two chromosomes. Such a person actually has genetic material equivalent to 47 chromosomes, even though the total number of chromosomes is not increased. A misplaced chromosome or part of a chromosome attached to another chromosome is called a *translocation* (*trans* = across + *locus* = place).

A large number of other clinical abnormalities have been described which are associated with trisomy of other chromosomes, chromosome translocation, or loss of entire chromosomes or portions of chromosomes.

CHROMOSOME ANALYSIS

The chromosome composition of the human cell can be studied with great accuracy and the presence of abnormalities in chromosome number or structure recognized. This can be accomplished by culturing human cells in a suitable medium. Usually human blood is used as a source of cells for these studies; the blood lymphocytes can be induced to undergo mitotic division. Certain chemicals are added which are capable of stopping the mitotic division after the chromosomes have become separate and distinct, so that many cells arrested in mitosis accumulate in the culture medium. Additional methods are employed to cause swelling of the cells, which increases the separation of the chromosomes. Then stained smears are prepared, and the chromosomes can be examined. Figure 11-1 (left) illustrates the appearance of a swollen cell arrested in mitosis with

Fig. 11-1.—Left, appearance of cell arrested in mitosis with chromosomes well separated. Right, individual chromosomes arranged in a standard pattern (karyotype).

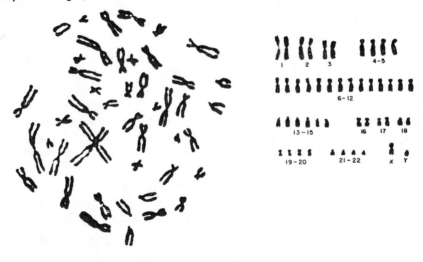

the chromosomes well separated. First, the spread chromosomes were photographed. Then, the individual chromosomes in the photograph were cut out and arranged according to size and the position of the central constriction, representing the site of attachment of the spindle fiber. Figure 11-1 (right) illustrates such a standard chromosome pattern, called a *karyotype*. The karyotype shown is from a normal male. A normal female pattern would be identical except for the presence of two X chromosomes rather than a single X and a single Y chromosome.

Congenital Abnormalities

Congenital abnormalities vary from minor deviations from normal to profound disturbances which are incompatible with extrauterine life. It is reported that, in 2 to 3 per cent of all live births, infants show one or more significant congenital abnormalities. However, some congenital abnormalities may not be identified at birth and become apparent only during the first year of life, so the actual incidence is probably even higher than 3 per cent. Three major categories of congenital abnormalities are recognized: (1) those due to abnormalities in the number and distribution of chromosomes, (2) those due to hereditary, genetically determined abnormalities of individual genes, and (3) those due to intrauterine injury to the developing fetus during a critical stage of development. Of the known congenital abnormalities, it has been estimated that approximately 10 per cent are due to intrauterine injury. Another 10 per cent are due to hereditary factors or abnormalities in chromosome number. In the remaining 80 per cent of cases, the exact cause of the congenital abnormality is unknown.

ABNORMALITIES OF THE CHROMOSOMES

Abnormalities in the distribution of chromosomes due to chromosome nondisjunction or translocation result in congenital defects. As has been discussed, the abnormalities may involve either autosomes or sex chromosomes. Mongolism is one of the more common conditions due to an autosomal abnormality. Several types of abnormalities involving sex chromosomes have also been described and are relatively common.

GENETICALLY DETERMINED DISEASES

Genetically determined diseases are the result of abnormalities of individual genes on the chromosome. The individual chromosomes appear normal, and the chromosome karyotype is normal. The genetic abnormality is transmitted from parent to offspring and may follow well-established mendelian inheritance patterns.

The genetic abnormality may be present on the sex chromosome (sex-linked inheritance) or on one of the other chromosomes (autosomal inheritance). Inheritance may follow a dominant pattern (disease transmitted by a single gene from either parent) or a recessive pattern (both parents must transmit an abnormal gene to the offspring). Many of the genetically determined diseases can be traced to a deficiency of a specific enzyme which is important in an intracellular metabolic reaction. Absence of the enzyme, resulting from abnormality of the gene, can produce profound disturbances in the cellular metabolic processes. Many different types of genetically determined cellular enzyme defects are recognized; these are sometimes called inborn errors of metabolism.

Figure 11-2 illustrates the sequence by which a genetic defect is translated into a specific disease. As indicated, a defective gene results in an absent or deficient enzyme within the cell. As a result of the enzyme de-

Fig. 11-2.—Mechanism by which a genetic defect is translated into a specific disease with characteristic clinical features.

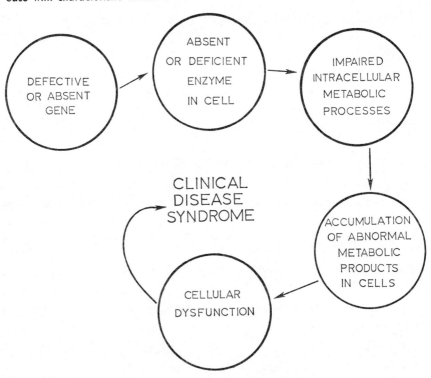

ficiency, enzyme-dependent metabolic processes are impaired. This, in turn, may lead to the accumulation of abnormal metabolic products within the cell, causing abnormalities in the function of the cell. The disturbed cell function is manifested to the physician as a disease with characteristic clinical features.

Developmental Abnormalities

Many sporadic abnormalities appear to be due to intrauterine injury during a critical stage of development. The injury may be due to maternal infection, to radiation, drugs, or unknown causes.

Maternal infections.—Certain infections acquired by the mother may injure the developing fetus. The most serious disease is German measles. If this infection develops during the first 4 weeks of pregnancy, congenital malformations occur in over half the infants born to affected mothers. However, this hazard exists only when the mother is susceptible to German measles. Of the adult population, 80 to 90 per cent is immune. Laboratory tests can determine whether a woman is susceptible to German measles.

Certain other viral infections and a few other kinds of maternal infection have also been shown to be capable of causing injury to the fetus. Fortunately, the great majority of infections acquired by the mother cause no congenital abnormalities.

Radiation.—Excessive radiation is a well-established cause of congenital abnormalities. Children born to Japanese women who were pregnant at the time of the atomic bomb explosions in World War II displayed a very high incidence of congenital abnormalities due to the injurious effect of radiation. Many other studies have also indicated that radiation is a hazard to the developing fetus.

Drugs.—Thalidomide, a tranquilizer and antiemetic compound, nas been shown to produce a high incidence of congenital abnormalities in the fetus when the drug is taken early in pregnancy. The most characteristic abnormality is partial or complete absence of the extremities, but other types of congenital abnormalities have also been produced. A few other drugs also have been implicated as a cause of congenital abnormalities. Because of the established relationship between congenital abnormalities and the ingestion of some drugs, most physicians recommend that the pregnant woman refrain from the indiscriminate use of drugs or other medications during the early part of pregnancy. Many new drugs and antibiotics are not recommended for use in pregnancy since their safety has not been established for pregnant women.

GENERAL PRINCIPLES REGARDING CONGENITAL ABNORMALITIES

In considering congenital abnormalities, one can make five generalizations:

(1) In the case of intrauterine injury due to drugs or other substances, the earlier in development the injury occurs the greater will be the ultimate effect on the developing fetus. A drug or virus infection may exert profound effects in the first few weeks of development but have little effect toward the end of pregnancy.

(2) Some major abnormalities, such as complete absence of a brain, heart, kidneys, or other vital structures may be compatible with normal intrauterine existence, even though such an abnormality is incompatible with life after delivery.

(3) Because of the complex developmental sequence involved in growth and differentiation, congenital abnormalities frequently involve multiple organ systems.

(4) Abnormalities in the development of one organ system are generally associated with an abnormal development of associated structures. For example, when the brain does not develop normally, frequently the overlying cranial cavity also does not develop in a normal manner.

(5) Congenital abnormalities frequently involve related organ systems which develop together. For example, the urinary system and the genital tract are related not only in physiologic function but also in their development. Therefore, it is quite common to find congenital abnormalities involving both organ systems. Since the heart and major blood vessel systems develop together, frequently congenital abnormalities involving the heart are associated with abnormalities in the vascular system as well.

PRENATAL DIAGNOSIS OF CONGENITAL ABNORMALITIES

Abnormalities induced by intrauterine injury occur sporadically and generally cannot be recognized prior to birth. However, many hereditary diseases which are associated with cellular enzyme deficiencies or accumulation of abnormal metabolic products within the cell and those associated with abnormalities in the numbers and distribution of chromosomes can be recognized by means of examination of cells obtained from amnionic fluid.

The cells in amnionic fluid are of fetal origin and are derived from fetal skin. The sex of the fetus can be determined by examining smears prepared from amnionic fluid for the presence of the sex chromatin body. More recently, it has been possible to culture amnionic cells in the laboratory by special technics and to determine the karyotype of the cells.

By this method, it has been possible to recognize mongolism and other abnormal conditions which are due to chromosome abnormalities. Amnionic fluid cells also contain many of the same metabolic enzymes present in the somatic cells of the fetus. Therefore, one can identify, by enzymatic analysis of cultured amnionic cells, many hereditary diseases which are associated with decrease or absence of intracellular enzyme systems.

Aspiration of amnionic fluid for diagnostic purposes (amniocentesis) is generally performed between the 14th and 18th week of pregnancy. This is advisable when the patient's family has a history of hereditary disease recognizable by amnionic cell study. The determination of fetal karyotype by this method has also been recommended in pregnancies of women over 38 to 40 years of age, since the incidence of mongolism is relatively high in the offspring of older women.

Chapter 12

Neoplasms

NORMAL LIFE PROCESSES are characterized by continuous growth and maturation of cells. This growth serves the purpose of replacing cells which have been injured or have undergone degenerative changes. In contrast, a neoplasm is an overgrowth of cells that serves no useful purpose. Neoplasms appear not to be subject to normal control mechanisms which regulate cell growth and differentiation.

The terms "neoplasm" and "tumor" have essentially the same meaning and may be used interchangeably. There are two large classes of neoplasms: benign tumors and malignant tumors.

Benign and Malignant Tumors

Generally a benign tumor grows slowly. The tumor remains localized, pushing aside surrounding normal tissue, but it does not infiltrate surrounding tissues or spread by blood and lymphatic channels to distant sites. Histologically, the cells in a benign tumor appear mature and closely resemble the normal cells from which the tumor was derived.

In contrast to the benign tumor, a malignant neoplasm grows more rapidly, infiltrating the surrounding tissues rather than growing in an expansile manner. Frequently, the infiltrating strands of tumor find their way into the vascular and lymphatic channels. Bits of tumor may be carried in the lymphatics to reach the lymph nodes, where they establish secondary sites of tumor growth not connected with the original tumor. Eventually the tumor may spread widely through the lymphatic channels. Tumor cells may also gain access to the blood stream and be carried to distant sites, leading to secondary tumor deposits throughout the body. The process by which a tumor spreads some distance from the primary site is called *metastasis* (*meta* = beyond + *stasis* = standing), and the secondary deposits are metastatic tumors. This property of metastasis is absent in benign tumors.

TABLE 12-1.—Comparison of Benign and Malignant Tumors

Characteristic	Benign Tumor	Malignant Tumor
Growth rate	Slow	Rapid
Character of growth	Expansion	Infiltration
Tumor spread	Remains localized	Metastasis by blood stream and lymphatics
Cell differentiation	Well differentiated	Poorly differentiated

Histologically, the cells of the malignant tumor are immature, being considerably less differentiated than the parent cells from which the tumors were derived. Table 12-1 summarizes the major differences between benign and malignant tumors.

Terminology

General Principles of Nomenclature

The terminology used in naming tumors is not completely uniform, but certain generalizations are possible. A benign tumor is frequently named from the tissue of origin, with the addition of the suffix "oma." Thus, a benign tumor of fibrous tissue is called a fibroma. A benign tumor of muscle is a myoma, and a benign tumor of glands is called an adenoma. (The root word for gland is "aden.")

There are many types of malignant tumors, each named according to the tissue of origin. For example, a malignant tumor derived from epithelium or glandular tissue is a carcinoma. A malignant tumor arising from the connective or supporting tissue is a sarcoma (*sarx* = flesh or muscle). The term sarcoma is also applied to neoplasms arising from reticuloendothelial and lymphoid tissue. A neoplasm of blood cells is called leukemia. The term "cancer" is a general word used to indicate any type of malignant tumor.

Malignant tumors are given additional names which further describe the cell from which the tumor developed. Thus, a carcinoma arising from squamous epithelium is a squamous cell carcinoma, and one arising from the transitional epithelium of the urinary bladder is a transitional cell carcinoma. A carcinoma arising from glands is an adenocarcinoma (*aden* = gland). Sarcomas are also designated by cell or tissue of origin. Thus, a malignant tumor of bone is an osteosarcoma. Myosarcoma develops from muscle; fibrosarcoma develops from connective tissue cells. A reticulum sarcoma develops from reticuloendothelial cells, and a lymphosarcoma develops from lymphoid tissue.

Variations in Terminology

There are some inconsistencies and exceptions to the general principles of nomenclature. Exceptions are encountered in the naming of lymphoid tumors, tumors of the pigment-producing cells, certain tumors of mixed cellular components, and certain types of embryonic tumors seen in children. Other examples will also be encountered where names of tumors seem to follow no rules or general principles. The student should not be unduly concerned about the exceptions or unusual situations, but rather should attempt to grasp general principles relating to the naming of tumors.

LYMPHOID TUMORS.—*Lymphoma* is the general term applied to all neoplasms of reticuloendothelial and lymphoid tissue. With extremely rare exceptions, these tumors are malignant. Therefore, the term lymphoma without qualification refers to a malignant, not a benign, tumor. Often, to avoid confusion, the term malignant lymphoma rather than simply lymphoma is used.

There are three main types of lymphoma: (1) reticulum cell sarcoma, arising from the reticuloendothelial tissues, (2) lymphosarcoma, from lymphoid tissue, and (3) Hodgkin's disease. Hodgkin's disease is a type of lymphoma which has a variable histologic appearance, consisting of large, neoplastic reticulum cells intermixed with lymphoid tissue and other cell types, and often associated with fibrous scarring.

TUMORS OF PIGMENT-PRODUCING EPITHELIUM.—The specialized pigment-producing cells in the skin which are responsible for normal skin color are called *nevus cells,* and the black pigment produced by the cells is called *melanin.* The common benign pigmented skin lesion is a *nevus,* the name being derived from the name of the cell. The malignant counterpart is called *melanoma* (or malignant melanoma), the name being derived from the pigment elaborated by the cells.

TUMORS OF MIXED COMPONENTS (TERATOMAS).—A teratoma is a tumor derived from cells which have the potential of differentiating into many different types of tissue (bone, muscle, glands, epithelium, brain tissue, hair) and frequently such tumors consist of poorly organized mixtures of many tissues. Tumors of this type often arise in the reproductive tract but may also occur in some other locations. Since a teratoma may be either benign or malignant, one must specify the type, calling the tumor either a benign teratoma or a malignant teratoma. A common type of cystic benign teratoma arising in the ovary is a *dermoid cyst.*

EMBRYONIC (EMBRYONAL) TUMORS.—Certain unusual tumors encountered in children are apparently derived from persisting groups of embryonic cells which have undergone neoplastic change. These tumors may arise in the brain, retina of the eye, adrenal gland, kidney, liver, or genital tract. Embryonic tumors of this type are named from the site of origin, with the suffix "blastoma" added (*blast* = a primitive cell, *oma* = tumor). Thus, an embryonic tumor arising from the medulla of the brain would be called a medulloblastoma. One arising from the retina of the eye is a retinoblastoma. An embryonic tumor of the kidney is called a nephroblastoma, and an embryonic tumor of hepatic origin would be called a hepatoblastoma.

Noninfiltrating (In Situ) Carcinoma

Infiltration and metastasis are two characteristic features of malignant tumors. However, we know now that many carcinomas arising from surface epithelium remain localized within the epithelium for many years before evidence of infiltration into the deeper tissues or spread to distant sites becomes apparent. This has been well documented in the case of squamous cell carcinoma of the cervix; noninfiltrating tumors have also been recognized in other locations. The term *carcinoma in situ* ("in site carcinoma") is used for this type of neoplasm. In situ carcinoma can be completely cured by surgical excision and is the most favorable stage for successful treatment.

Incidence and Survival Rates in Patients with Malignant Tumors

Malignant neoplasms are a leading cause of disability and death. Cancer is second only to heart disease as a cause of death in the United States, accounting for almost 17 per cent of all deaths in this country. It has been estimated that one in every four individuals will eventually develop cancer. Of the cancers involving major organs, lung carcinoma is the most common malignant tumor in men, and breast carcinoma is the most frequent in women. Carcinoma of the intestine is also quite common in both sexes. The survival rate for patients with malignant tumors depends on early diagnosis and treatment, before the disease has spread. The chances for survival are markedly reduced if the tumor has metastasized to regional lymph nodes or distant sites.

Cytologic Diagnosis of Neoplasms

Tumors shed abnormal cells from their surfaces, and these cells can be recognized in the body fluids and secretions that come into contact with the tumor. Often the abnormal cells can be recognized when the neoplasm is only microscopic in size and still confined to the surface epithelium. These observations have been applied to the cytologic diagnosis of tumors. The method is named after the physician who played a large part in developing and applying cytologic methods, Dr. George Papanicolaou. The microscopic slides of the material prepared for cytologic examination are called *Papanicolaou smears,* or simply "Pap smears."

In carcinoma of the uterine cervix, abnormal cells can often be found in the vaginal secretions. Widespread application of the cytologic method has led to much earlier detection of cervical carcinoma than was possible previously. Indeed, it has played a significant role in reducing the mortality from carcinoma of the uterine cervix. Cytologic methods can also be applied to the diagnosis of neoplasms in other locations by means of examining sputum, urine, breast secretions, and fluids obtained from the pleural or peritoneal cavity. However, the greatest usefulness of the method has been in the early diagnosis of cervical cancer.

It should be emphasized that an abnormal Pap smear indicates only that the epithelium is shedding abnormal cells. It does not necessarily indicate a diagnosis of cancer, since occasionally some benign diseases may also be associated with the desquamation of atypical cells. A Pap smear should be considered a screening procedure, and an abnormal smear should always be followed by a biopsy and histologic examination of the tissue, in order to establish an exact diagnosis.

Leukemia

The term *leukemia* refers to a neoplasm of hematopoietic tissue. In contrast to solid tumors, which form nodular deposits, leukemic cells diffusely infiltrate the bone marrow and lymphoid tissues, spill over into the bloodstream, and infiltrate throughout the various organs of the body. The leukemic cells may be mostly mature cells or they may be extremely primitive. The overproduction of white cells in leukemia may be reflected in the peripheral blood by a very high white blood count. However, in some cases of leukemia, the proliferation of the white cells is largely confined to the bone marrow, and there is no significant increase in the number of white cells in the blood stream.

CLASSIFICATION OF LEUKEMIA

Leukemia is classified on the basis of both the cell type and the maturity of the proliferating cells. Any type of hematopoietic cell can give rise to leukemia, but the most common types are granulocytic, monocytic, and lymphocytic. Leukemia developing from stem cells which would normally give rise to the leukocytes containing specific granules (neutrophils, eosinophils, and basophils) is called granulocytic leukemia. Monocytic leukemia develops from precursor cells which give rise to monocytes. Lymphocytic leukemia is derived from lymphoid precursor cells.

If the leukemia cells are mostly primitive forms, the leukemia is classified as acute leukemia. In chronic leukemia, the abnormal cells are mostly mature cells.

In most instances, the total number of white blood cells in the peripheral blood is markedly elevated above normal. However, occasionally the marrow may be crowded with abnormal cells, but the number of white blood cells in the blood is normal or decreased. This variety of leukemia is sometimes called aleukemic leukemia. This is merely a descriptive term and does not denote a type of leukemia with any special clinical features or any difference in prognosis.

Generally, the classifications by cell type and maturity are used together. Thus, one may speak of chronic granulocytic leukemia, acute lymphocytic leukemia, acute monocytic leukemia, etc. The term "aleukemic" is often added if the number of white cells in the circulating blood is reduced.

CLINICAL FEATURES OF LEUKEMIA

The clinical features of leukemia are of two types, those due to impairment of bone marrow function and those due to infiltration of the viscera by leukemic cells. The overgrowth of leukemic cells in the bone marrow often crowds out normal bone marrow cells. This leads to anemia due to inadequate red cell production, bleeding due to thrombocytopenia, and infection resulting from inadequate numbers of normal white blood cells which are an important part of the body's defenses against pathogenic organisms.

The leukemic cells not only infiltrate the bone marrow but also spread into the spleen, liver, lymph nodes, and other tissues. In chronic leukemia, the evolution of the disease proceeds at a relatively slow pace and often can be well controlled by treatment for long periods of time. Therefore, the patient with chronic leukemia may survive for many years in relatively good health. In contrast, acute leukemia is a rapidly progressive disease. Symptoms of bone marrow infiltration and visceral infiltration make their appearance early and are quite conspicuous. Death may follow within a few months. In some patients with acute leukemia, the abnormal proliferation of the leukemic cells can be stopped for a variable period of time by certain drugs and chemicals, and the patient appears to have completely recovered. An arrest of the disease induced by therapy is called a remission. However, eventually the patient undergoes a relapse and the disease ultimately proves fatal.

Multiple Myeloma

Multiple myeloma is a neoplasm arising from plasma cells within the bone marrow. In many ways, it resembles leukemia. However, the neoplastic plasma cell proliferation is generally confined to the bone marrow. Infiltration of the viscera by the abnormal plasma cells is unusual; outpouring of large numbers of plasma cells into the peripheral blood is also uncommon. The abnormal plasma cells may either infiltrate the bone marrow diffusely or form discrete tumors which weaken the bone, leading to spontaneous fractures, pain, and disability. Normal plasma cells produce antibody proteins. In myeloma, the neoplastic cells also often produce large amounts of protein. This markedly increases blood proteins and, correspondingly, blood viscosity. The myeloma protein differs from the protein normally found in the blood and can be identified in a patient's blood by various special laboratory technics. Masses of coagulated myeloma protein may accumulate within the patient's own tissues and cause marked impairment of the function of the involved tissues. Some patients with myeloma die of kidney failure resulting from infiltration of the kidneys and obstruction of the kidney tubules by masses of protein produced by the plasma cells.

Early Recognition of Neoplasms

The American Cancer Society lists a number of signs and symptoms which should arouse suspicion of cancer. In general, any abnormality of form or function may be an early symptom of a neoplasm and should be investigated by a physician. For example, a lump in the breast, an ulcer on the lip, or a change in the character of a wart or mole may be considered an abnormality of form. Irregular menstrual bleeding in a postmenopausal woman or a change in bowel habits manifested by constipation or diarrhea is an abnormality of function.

A complete medical history and physical examination by the physician are the next steps in evaluating suspected abnormalities. The physical examination may include special studies, such as an examination of the rectum and colon by means of a special instrument, vaginal examination and Pap smear in women, examination of the esophagus and stomach with special devices, and various types of x-ray studies.

If a tumor is discovered, exact diagnosis requires biopsy or complete excision of the suspected tumor. Histologic examination of the tissue by the pathologist will provide an exact diagnosis and serve as a guide to further treatment. If the tumor is benign, simple excision is curative. If the tumor is malignant, a more extensive operation or other type of treatment may be required.

Frozen Section Diagnosis of Neoplasms

Many times it is important that the surgeon learn immediately whether a tumor he has found during operation is benign or malignant, because the type of surgery performed may depend on the nature of the neoplasm. Often, the surgeon must also find out during the operation whether a tumor has been excised completely or whether it has spread to lymph nodes or distant sites. The pathologist can provide him with a rapid histologic diagnosis and other information by means of a special technic called a *frozen section*. In this method, a portion of the tumor or other tissue to be examined histologically is frozen solid at subzero temperature. A thin section of the frozen tissue is cut by means of a special instrument called a microtome, and slides are prepared and stained. The slides can then be examined by the pathologist and a rapid histologic diagnosis can be made. The entire procedure takes only a few minutes.

Treatment of Neoplasms

Benign tumors are completely cured by surgical excision. Most malignant tumors are treated by wide surgical excision of the tumor and surrounding tissues, often with removal of the regional lymph nodes which drain the tumor site. This is often successful if the tumor has not already metastasized to distant sites. If the tumor is too widespread for surgical attack, x-ray therapy may be used to control the tumor, but usually it is not curative. Some malignant tumors can be controlled temporarily by hormone therapy or by means of various drugs. Lymphoid tissue is extremely susceptible to radiation, and x-ray therapy is generally used to treat malignant lymphomas of all types. Leukemia is treated by various drugs and chemicals which impede the growth of the leukemic cells. Some types of leukemia respond to adrenal corticosteroid therapy.

Viruses and Neoplasms

Many types of tumors in animals are due to viruses and can be readily transmitted by appropriate methods to animals of the same or different species. In some instances, a single type of virus is capable of producing many different types of tumors in various species of animals. At least some of the cancers in humans also appear to be due to viruses.

Immunologic Defenses Against Neoplasms

The actual cause of cancer is unknown. However, the basic process is an alteration in the chromosomes of the cell, so that the cell no longer responds to normal control mechanisms and is capable of independent growth unrelated to the needs of the body. An alteration in cell chromosomes is called a *mutation* (*muto* = change).

In the body, many billions of cells are dividing repeatedly. They are continually subjected to influences which disturb the process of normal cell division and may lead to the formation of abnormal cells. For example, a virus may enter a cell and alter its genetic structure by becoming incorporated into the nucleoprotein of the cell chromosomes. Radiation and various chemical carcinogens (cancer-producing substances) may also induce mutation by altering chromosome structure. Probably many other factors can also influence the dividing cell. Sometimes more than one agent may be necessary to produce a transformation of the cell, whereas one alone would be harmless. For example, a carcinogen may activate a latent virus; the cell mutation induced would reflect the combined effect of both virus and chemical agent.

The mutant cell differs from the normal cell and contains new antigens not present in the normal cell. The abnormal cell, no longer subject to normal control mechanisms, begins to proliferate, and unchecked proliferation leads to the development of a tumor. However, the body recognizes the new antigens in the abnormal cell as foreign antigens and attempts to destroy the cell by means of the various cellular and humoral defense mechanisms which have been described previously.

Apparently mutations leading to neoplastic transformation of cells are relatively common, but the body recognizes the altered cells as abnormal and destroys them as soon as they are formed. Only a tiny proportion of abnormal cells ever develop into clinically apparent tumors. Therefore, a tumor may be considered to represent a failure of the body's immune defenses. There is support for this concept, since individuals with congenital deficiencies of immunologic defense mechanisms have a high incidence of tumors. This is also true of persons whose immune responses have been deliberately suppressed by drugs or other substances.

Figure 12-1 illustrates the interrelationship of the factors concerned with the defenses against tumors. On the one hand, abnormal cells arise and tend to proliferate, leading to tumors. On the other hand, the immune defense mechanisms destroy these abnormal cells before they can prove hazardous to the body. Tumors result when the defense mechanisms fail. Fortunately, in most instances the immune surveillance system eliminates the "bad" cells as soon as they appear. Although the immune de-

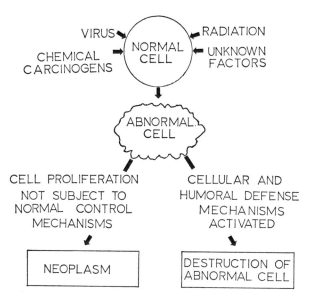

Fig. 12-1.—Factors leading to neoplastic transformation of cells counterbalanced by immunologic defenses against neoplasm.

fense mechanisms are quite efficient in eliminating abnormal cells before they develop into a tumor, they are relatively ineffective in eliminating an established tumor. For this reason, attempts to treat tumors by "vaccines" prepared from tumor cells or by other immunologic methods have been unsuccessful.

Chapter 13

Abnormalities of Blood Coagulation

IF ONE CUTS a finger with a knife, tne cut bleeds, put the bleeding soon stops and healing ensues. The body has a complex mechanism for causing blood to clot when it is necessary, while at the same time maintaining the blood in a fluid state within the capillaries and larger blood vessels.

The proper function of the hemostatic mechanism depends upon the interaction of a number of factors: the integrity of the small blood vessels, normal numbers of blood platelets, normal amounts of plasma coagulation factors, and normal concentrations of inhibitors of blood coagulation. If any one of these is abnormal, the blood coagulation mechanism will not function properly. Adequate levels of calcium are also required for normal blood coagulation. However, no diseases are known in which disturbances of blood coagulation are due to abnormal levels of serum calcium.

The process of blood coagulation may be considered as a chain reaction in which each component in the chain is formed from an inactive precursor present in the blood, and each activated component in turn activates the next member of the chain in a sequential manner. It is somewhat analogous to knocking over the first in a long chain of dominoes. Tipping the first domino corresponds to the initiation of the clotting mechanism. The fall of the last domino represents the formation of a firm blood clot.

Although blood coagulation is actually a continuous sequence, the clotting mechanism is arbitrarily divided into three stages for descriptive purposes (Fig. 13-1). The first phase concerns the formation of thromboplastin; it may be initiated by either of two separate mechanisms. One mechanism depends on the interaction of platelets and plasma coagulation factors. If the wall of a blood vessel is injured, platelets accumulate at the

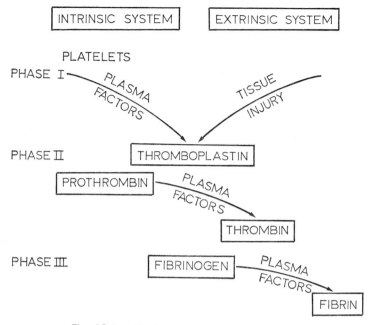

Fig. 13-1.—Mechanism of blood coagulation.

site and liberate various components which react with plasma factors to form thromboplastin. This is called the *intrinsic system* of thromboplastin formation, since the thromboplastin is produced from substances present within the bloodstream. However, many tissues also have thromboplastic activity, and tissue injury liberates substances from them. This is called the *extrinsic system* of thromboplastin formation, because the thromboplastin is derived not from the bloodstream but from tissues extrinsic to the vascular compartment.

The second phase of coagulation concerns the conversion of prothrombin to thrombin. Additional plasma coagulation factors are necessary for this step. The third phase is concerned with the conversion of fibrinogen to fibrin. Still other plasma factors are required in this phase for stabilizing and strengthening the fibrin clot. The fibrin clot entraps white cells, platelets, and red cells, forming a gelatinous plug which represents the end stage of the clotting process.

In addition to coagulation factors, a number of other substances in the plasma act as physiologic inhibitors of blood coagulation. Another factor called *fibrinolysin* (*lysis* = dissolving) is capable of dissolving the fibrin in blood clots. These substances probably function by restricting the clotting process to a limited area, thereby preventing excessive or uncontrolled intravascular clotting.

Clinical Disturbances of Blood Coagulation

Disturbances of blood coagulation may be classified in one of four large categories: (1) abnormalities of small blood vessels, (2) abnormalities of platelet numbers or platelet function, (3) deficiency of one or more of the plasma coagulation factors, and (4) liberation of thromboplastic material into the circulation.

ABNORMALITIES OF THE SMALL BLOOD VESSELS

Some rare diseases characterized by abnormal bleeding have been found to be due to abnormal function of the small blood vessels. Normally, small blood vessels contract after injury, helping seal the defect by a blood clot. Sometimes this function is defective, leading to excessive bleeding. There are a few other diseases in which the small blood vessels are abnormally formed and cannot function properly.

ABNORMALITIES OF PLATELET NUMBERS OR FUNCTION

A decrease in platelets is called thrombocytopenia (*thrombus* = clot + *cyte* = cell + *penia* = deficiency). This may be due to injury or disease of the bone marrow, which damages the megakaryocytes in the marrow, the precursor cells of the platelets. Thrombocytopenia may also be due to antiplatelet autoantibodies which cause destruction of the platelets in the peripheral blood (as seen in some autoimmune diseases). Sometimes platelets are normal in number but abnormal in function, so that they are ineffective in initiating the clotting process.

Bleeding associated with defective or inadequate platelets is generally manifested by small, pinpoint areas of bleeding in skin and deeper tissues (called petechiae or petechial hemorrhages) rather than by large areas of hemorrhage.

DEFICIENCY OF THE PLASMA COAGULATION FACTORS

A deficiency of a single plasma factor concerned in the first stage of coagulation is usually hereditary. Hemophilia is the best-known example of a hereditary coagulation factor deficiency. This is a sex-linked recessive abnormality characterized by defective synthesis of antihemophiliac globulin.

Abnormalities in the second phase of coagulation are due to a deficiency of prothrombin or other factors required for the conversion of prothrombin to thrombin. These factors are synthesized in the liver. Vitamin K is required for the synthesis of most of these substances (called vitamin-K-dependent factors). Impaired blood coagulation due to decreased levels of these factors is usually due either to administration of anticoagulant drugs or to severe liver disease. Anticoagulant drugs are sometimes used to treat patients who have an increased tendency to develop intravascular thrombosis. They are also administered to patients with some types of heart disease. Many of these drugs act by inhibiting the synthesis of vitamin-K-dependent clotting factors by the liver. Their effect can be counteracted by the administration of vitamin K. Patients with severe liver disease may also have disturbances of blood coagulation because the liver has been so badly damaged that synthesis of adequate levels of coagulation factors is no longer possible.

LIBERATION OF THROMBOPLASTIC MATERIAL INTO THE CIRCULATION

In a number of diseases associated with shock, overwhelming bacterial infection, or extensive necrosis of tissue, products of tissue necrosis and other substances with thromboplastic activity are liberated into the circulation, leading to widespread intravascular coagulation of the blood. In the process of clotting, platelets and the various plasma coagulation factors are utilized, and the levels of these components in the blood drop precipitously.

The body's defense against widespread intravascular clotting consists of activation of the fibrinolysin system; this dissolves clots and prevents potentially lethal obstruction of the circulatory system by massive intravascular coagulation. The breakdown products produced from the degradation of the fibrin act as additional inhibitors of the clotting process.

The net effect of these various events is a bleeding disturbance, sometimes in a patient already seriously ill because of an underlying disease which caused activation of the blood-clotting mechanism. This abnormal bleeding state is called *disseminated intravascular coagulation*, or *consumption coagulopathy*. The latter term alludes to the consumption of the clotting factors as a result of the pathologic coagulation process.

Chapter 14

Circulatory Disturbances

Thrombosis and Embolism

NORMALLY BLOOD does not clot within the vascular system. However, under unusual circumstances, intravascular clotting may occur due to (1) slowing or stasis of the blood flow, (2) damage to the wall of the blood vessel, and/or (3) increase in the coagulability of the blood. Frequently more than one factor is responsible for intravascular clotting.

An intravascular clot is called a *thrombus;* the condition is termed *thrombosis.* Intravascular thrombi may form within veins, arteries, and occasionally within the heart itself. A clot in the vascular system may become detached and be carried in the circulation. Such a clot is termed an *embolus* (*embolus* = plug or stopper); the condition is termed *embolism.* Depending upon where the blood clot was formed initially, the embolus may be carried into either the pulmonary or systemic arterial circulation. Eventually, it is arrested in an artery of smaller caliber than the diameter of the clot. When the embolus plugs the vessel, it blocks the blood flow to the tissue distal to the obstruction, and the damaged tissue may undergo necrosis if the collateral blood supply is inadequate. The area of tissue breakdown is called an *infarct* or *infarction.*

VENOUS THROMBOSIS

Formation of blood clots within leg veins is usually due primarily to slowing or stasis of the blood in the veins. This is likely to occur during periods of prolonged bed rest, or after a cramped position is maintained for a long period of time. Under these circumstances, the normal "milking action" of the leg musculature, promoting venous return, is impaired, leading to stasis of the blood. Varicose veins or any condition preventing normal emptying of veins predisposes an individual to thrombosis by causing venous stasis.

Postoperative thrombosis in leg veins is a common problem. The effects of the venous stasis resulting from inactivity combined with increased blood coagulability (due to an increased concentration of blood coagulation factors) make surgical patients susceptible to venous thrombosis.

A venous thrombosis may partially block venous return in the leg, making the leg swell. However, the major complication of venous thrombosis is related to detachment of the clot from the wall of the vein. A venous thrombosis which breaks loose is carried into the pulmonary circulation, and the embolus may block the main pulmonary artery, causing sudden death because of complete obstruction of blood flow to the lungs. A smaller embolus may be carried into a branch of the pulmonary artery, causing an infarction of the portion of the lung supplied by the occluded vessel. The area of infarction is characterized by necrosis of the walls of the pulmonary alveoli and alveolar capillaries, leading to leakage of blood into the damaged portion of lung. Blood from the hemorrhagic infarcted area often appears in the bronchial secretions, and the patient with a pulmonary infarct may cough up blood-streaked sputum. The patient also frequently experiences chest pain because of inflammation of the pleura overlying the infarct.

ARTERIAL THROMBOSIS

Blood flow in arteries is rapid and intravascular pressure is high, so that stasis of blood is not a factor in arterial thrombosis. The main cause of arterial thrombosis is injury to the wall of the vessel, usually secondary to arteriosclerosis. The arteriosclerotic deposits cause ulceration and roughening of the lining of the artery, and thrombi form on the roughened area. The effects of arterial thrombus formation depend upon the location and size of the artery which has become obstructed. Blockage of a coronary artery frequently causes infarction of the heart muscle, and consequent "heart attack." If a major artery supplying the leg is occluded, the extremity undergoes necrosis, usually called *gangrene*. (This differs from gas gangrene, which is caused by a species of *Clostridium*.) Occlusion of an artery to the brain leads to infarction of a portion of the brain, commonly called a "stroke."

INTRACARDIAC THROMBOSIS

Occasionally blood clots may form within the heart itself. Thrombi may form within the atrial appendages when heart function is abnormal, as in heart failure, or when the atria are not contracting normally. Thrombi may also form on the surfaces of heart valves which have been damaged as a result of disease. Occasionally, thrombi may form on the internal lining of the ventricle adjacent to an area of infarction of heart muscle. Intracardiac thrombi may become dislodged and carried into the systemic circulation, resulting in infarction of spleen, kidney, brain, or other organs. The symptoms produced depend upon the size and location of the infarction.

Thrombosis Due to Increased Blood Coagulability

In some conditions, the concentrations of various blood coagulation factors are elevated; this increases the coagulability of the blood and predisposes the individual to intravascular clotting. After injury or operation, products of tissue necrosis stimulate the synthesis of many clotting factors, increasing the likelihood of postoperative thrombosis in leg veins (discussed previously).

Recently, the estrogen in contraceptive pills has been found to increase the concentration of many blood clotting factors, predisposing the women who use them to both venous and arterial thrombosis. This observation has led to concern about the safety of "the pill" when used for long periods of time.

Men with prostatic carcinoma are sometimes treated with estrogen to cause regression of the tumor. Sometimes this treatment is complicated by intravascular thrombosis, due to the effect of large doses of estrogen.

Embolism Due to Foreign Material

Most emboli are due to blood clots. However, occasionally other materials gain access to the circulation. Fat, air, and foreign particles within the vascular system may sometimes cause serious difficulties.

FAT EMBOLISM.—After a severe bone fracture, fatty bone marrow and surrounding adipose tissue may be disrupted. The emulsified fat globules may be sucked into the veins and carried into the lungs, leading to widespread obstruction of the pulmonary capillaries. Some of the fat may be carried through the pulmonary capillaries and reach the systemic circulation, eventually blocking small blood vessels in the brain and other organs.

AIR EMBOLISM.—Sometimes a large amount of air is sucked into the venous circulation after a chest wound involving lung injury. Air may also be accidentally injected into the circulation during attempts at abortion by persons without medical training. The air is carried to the heart and accumulates in the right heart chambers, preventing filling of the heart by returning venous blood. As a result, the heart is unable to pump blood, and the individual dies rapidly of circulatory failure.

Embolism of particulate foreign material.—Various types of particulate material may be injected into veins by drug addicts. The material is usually trapped within the small pulmonary blood vessels, producing symptoms of severe respiratory distress due to obstruction of the pulmonary capillaries by the foreign material.

Edema

Edema refers to accumulation of fluid in the interstitial tissues. Edema is most conspicuous in the skin and subcutaneous tissues of the dependent parts of the body and is usually noted first in the legs and ankles. When the edematous tissue is compressed by indenting the tissue with the fingertips, the fluid is pushed aside, leaving a pit or indentation which gradually refills with fluid. This characteristic is responsible for the common term "pitting edema." Fluid may also accumulate in the pleural cavity (*hydrothorax*) or in the peritoneal cavity (*ascites*).

Edema may result from any condition in which the circulation of extracellular fluid between the capillaries and the interstitial tissues becomes disturbed.

Factors Regulating Flow of Fluid Between Capillaries and Interstitial Tissues

Flow of fluid in and out of capillaries depends on several factors. Osmotic pressure is the force which tends to hold fluid within the capillaries. This may be defined as the property causing fluid to migrate in the direction of a higher concentration of molecules. The osmotic pressure of the plasma depends primarily on the concentration of the plasma proteins. Since the capillaries are impermeable to protein, the protein tends to draw water from the interstitial fluid into the capillaries and to hold it there. The plasma osmotic pressure depends mostly on the number of molecules and not on the size of the molecules. Albumin exerts a greater osmotic effect than globulin, because the albumin molecule is a much smaller molecule than are globulin molecules. Therefore, there are more molecules per gram of albumin than per gram of globulins.

The osmotic effect of the plasma protein is counterbalanced by the hydrostatic pressure. This is the pressure of the blood within the capillaries which tends to push fluid out of the capillaries. The hydrostatic pressure exceeds the plasma osmotic pressure at the arterial end of the capillaries, and fluid tends to leave the vessels. At the venous end of the capillaries, the hydrostatic pressure is lower, so that fluid tends to diffuse back into the capillaries. As a consequence of this circulation, dissolved nutrients are carried from the blood into the interstitial tissues to nourish the cells, and waste products are returned to the circulation for excretion. Some fluid forced out of the capillaries by the hydrostatic pressure of the blood does not diffuse back into the capillaries but returns to the circulation via lymphatic channels.

PATHOGENESIS AND CLASSIFICATION OF EDEMA

Edema is classified on the basis of the primary factor responsible for the accumulation of fluid. Four major causes of edema are recognized: (1) increased capillary permeability, (2) low plasma proteins, (3) increased hydrostatic pressure, and (4) lymphatic obstruction.

INCREASED CAPILLARY PERMEABILITY.—Increased capillary permeability allows transudation of excess fluid from the capillaries. The localized edema associated with an acute inflammation is due to increased capillary permeability. Some systemic diseases are also associated with altered capillary permeability, leading to generalized edema.

LOW PLASMA PROTEINS.—Plasma osmotic pressure is reduced if plasma proteins are decreased. Plasma proteins may be lost in the urine due to glomerular injury, or their synthesis may be impaired due to malnutrition. Hypoproteinemia due to malnutrition may be encountered in patients with various types of chronic debilitating disease who are unable to eat adequate amounts of food, or in patients with various types of chronic intestinal disease, in whom assimilation of food is impaired.

INCREASED HYDROSTATIC PRESSURE.—High venous pressure causes high capillary pressure, leading to excessive transudation of fluid from the capillaries. This situation is encountered most frequently as a manifestation of heart failure. Occasionally, elevated venous pressure may be due to an obstruction of a vein, as by a venous thrombosis, resulting in localized edema of the tissues distal to the site of obstruction.

LYMPHATIC OBSTRUCTION.—Some of the fluid which normally escapes from the capillaries is returned to the circulation via lymphatic channels. If the lymphatic drainage of a part of the body is obstructed, edema may develop in the area drained by the obstructed lymphatic channels. Sometimes this happens after certain types of surgical operations. In the treatment of carcinoma of the breast, a radical operation is performed in which the axillary lymph nodes and axillary tissues are resected along with the breast. Sometimes the axilla is also subjected to radiation therapy. These procedures may cause obstruction of the lymphatic drainage from the upper arm, which also drains into the axilla, resulting in edema of the arm. Obstruction of inguinal lymph nodes due to various diseases may also occasionally cause pronounced edema of the lower extremity.

Chapter 15

The Cardiovascular System

THE HEART is a muscular pump which propels blood through the lungs and to the peripheral tissues. Heart disease is due to a disturbance in the function of the cardiac pump. A working knowledge of the normal structure and function of the heart is essential to an understanding of the various types of heart disease.

Normal Cardiac Function

CARDIAC CHAMBERS

The heart is divided by partitions into four chambers, the right and left atria and the right and left ventricles. No direct communication exists between the right and left halves of the heart, and it is convenient clinically to consider each half of the heart as an independent structure. The "right heart" circulates blood into the pulmonary artery and through the lungs (the pulmonary circulation); the "left heart" pumps blood into the aorta for distribution to the various organs and tissues of the body (the systemic circulation).

CARDIAC VALVES

The flow of blood in and out of the cardiac chambers is controlled by a system of valves which normally permit flow in only one direction. The atrioventricular valves are flap-like valves surrounding the orifices between atria and ventricles. The free margins of the valves are connected to the walls of the ventricles by narrow, string-like bands of fibrous tissue, the *chordae tendineae*. The semilunar valves, surrounding the orifices of the aorta and pulmonary artery, are positioned so that the free margins of the valves face upward. This structural arrangement defines cup-like pockets between the free margins of the valves and the roots of the blood vessels to which the valves are attached.

When the heart relaxes in diastole, the chordae produce tension on the valves and pull the atrioventricular valves apart. When the ventricles contract, the chordae are no longer under tension, and the force of the blood flow pushes the valves together, so that no blood flows from the ventricles into the atria. During ventricular contraction, the semilunar valves are forced apart by the jets of blood leaving the ventricles. When ventricular contraction ceases, the weight of the column of ejected blood forces the valves back into position, preventing reflux of blood into the ventricles during diastole. The atrioventricular and semilunar valves function in a reciprocal manner. Ventricular contraction relaxes tension on the chordae, resulting in closure of the atrioventricular valves at the same time that the jets of blood open the semilunar valves. Closure of the semilunar valves in diastole is also associated with opening of the atrioventricular valves. Figure 15-1 illustrates the reciprocal action of the two sets of valves, which is responsible for the unidirectional flow required for normal cardiac function.

BLOOD SUPPLY TO THE HEART

The heart is supplied by two large *coronary arteries* which arise from the aortic sinuses at the root of the aorta.

BLOOD PRESSURE

The flow of blood in the arteries is due to the force of ventricular contraction. The pressure within the arteries varies rhythmically with the beating of the heart. The highest pressure is reached during the ventricular contraction (systolic pressure); the pressure is lowest when the ventricles are relaxed (diastolic pressure). The peripheral arterioles regulate the rate of blood flow into the capillaries by varying the degree of arteriolar constriction. In many respects, the effect is analogous to the resistance to outflow of water from a garden hose, which can be varied by tightening or loosening the nozzle on the hose. Because of the resistance offered by the arterioles, the blood pressure during cardiac diastole does not fall to zero, but declines slowly as blood leaves the large arteries through the arterioles into the capillaries.

In summary, the systolic blood pressure is a measure of the force of ventricular contraction as blood is ejected into the large arteries. The diastolic pressure is a measure of the rate of "run-off" of blood into the capillaries, which is governed by the peripheral resistance due to the small arterioles throughout the body. The mean (average) pressure of blood in the large arteries is midway between systolic and diastolic pressure.

SYSTOLE   DIASTOLE

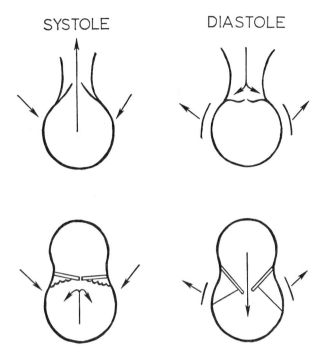

Fig. 15-1.—Reciprocal action of atrioventricular and semilunar valves, resulting in unidirectional blood flow.

Heart Disease as a Disturbance of Pump Function

For a pump to function properly, several conditions are required:

(1) The pump must be properly constructed so that it is free of mechanical defects.

(2) The pump must have a system of valves to permit unidirectional flow. If valves do not function properly, the force of the pump stroke is dissipated and effective pumping is impaired.

(3) The pump must have an adequate fuel supply. It will not run properly if the fuel mixture is too lean or if the fuel line is plugged.

(4) The pump must be used within its rated capacity. One must not use a pump rated at 3 horsepower to perform a job requiring a 10-horsepower pump. Either the pump will not function at all, or it will wear out very rapidly.

The heart is subject to the requirements of any mechanical pump. Each of the various types of heart disease can be considered to correspond to one of the derangements indicated above which would impair the function of any mechanical pump. Congenital heart disease corresponds to faulty pump construction. Rheumatic heart disease can be equated with abnormalities in the valve system of a pump. Arteriosclerotic heart disease is comparable to pump failure due to inadequate fuel supply. Heart disease due to high blood pressure can be compared to overloading a pump by using it in excess of its rated capacity.

CONGENITAL HEART DISEASE

The heart undergoes a complicated developmental sequence. It is formed by fusion of paired tubes. The fused cardiac tube undergoes segmental dilatations and constrictions, along with marked growth and change in configuration. Eventually, the individual chambers, valves, and large arteries develop, leading to the final structural configuration of the normal heart.

Sometimes the heart fails to develop normally. This may result in defective communication between cardiac chambers, malformation of cardiac valves or septa, or malformation of the large vessels entering and leaving the cardiac chambers. Some virus infections, especially German measles in the mother during the early phases of fetal development, may cause improper development of the heart, as well as other organs. Some chromosomal abnormalities, such as mongolism, are also frequently associated with abnormal cardiac development. In many instances, the reason for congenital heart abnormalities cannot be determined.

The effect of a structural abnormality depends on the nature of the defect. Some congenital abnormalities can be corrected relatively easily by various types of surgical operations. Some cannot be corrected by surgery but may be compatible with a relatively normal life. Still others cause serious malfunction of the heart and are rapidly fatal in the neonatal period.

PREVENTION.—The only way to prevent congenital heart disease is to attempt to protect the developing fetus from intrauterine injury during the early phases of pregnancy when it is extremely vulnerable. The various factors that may cause intrauterine fetal injury have been discussed in the section on congenital abnormalities (Chapter 11).

RHEUMATIC FEVER

Rheumatic fever is a complication of an infection by the beta hemolytic streptococcus, the organism responsible for streptococcal sore throat and scarlet fever. This disease, encountered most commonly in children, is a febrile illness associated with inflammation of connective tissue throughout the body, especially in the heart and joints. Clinically, the affected individual has an acute arthritis involving multiple joints (which is why the disease is called "rheumatic" fever) and evidence of inflammation of the heart.

Rheumatic fever is not a bacterial infection, but a manifestation of a hypersensitivity state caused by various antigens present in the streptococcus. This state develops several weeks after the initial streptococcal infection. It is uncertain exactly how the streptococcus induces the development of rheumatic fever. Apparently, some persons form antibody against antigens present in the streptococcus, and the antistreptococcal antibody cross-reacts with similar antigens in the individual's own tissues. The antigen-antibody reaction injures connective tissue and is responsible for the febrile illness. Fortunately, rheumatic fever develops in only a small proportion of persons with streptococcal infections.

Some patients with acute rheumatic fever die as a result of severe inflammation of the heart and consequent acute heart failure. However, in most instances, the fever and signs of inflammation eventually subside. Healing is often associated with some degree of scarring. In the joints and many other tissues, scarring causes no difficulties, but scarring of heart valves may produce various deformities which impair their proper function.

Unfortunately, a person who has had rheumatic fever is prone to recurrent rheumatic fever when he develops another streptococcal infection, since any subsequent contact with the streptococcus reestablishes the sequence of hypersensitivity and connective tissue damage.

RHEUMATIC HEART DISEASE

Rheumatic heart disease is a complication of rheumatic fever. It results from scarring of the heart valves subsequent to the healing of a rheumatic inflammation of the valves. This is a relatively common complication and involves primarily the valves of the left side of the heart, the mitral and aortic valves. If the valve does not close properly, blood refluxes back through it (called *regurgitation*). Frequently the damaged valve also does not open properly, and the valve orifice is narrowed. This is called a valve *stenosis*. Valve lesions impair normal cardiac function. In a valvular stenosis, the heart must exert more effort than normal to force blood through the narrowed orifice. In regurgitation, a proportion of the ventricular output is not expelled normally and leaks through the incompetent valve. This is a serious disadvantage, since the heart must repump the volume of regurgitated blood to deliver the same amount of blood to the peripheral tissues.

The individual with a mild rheumatic valvular deformity which does not interfere seriously with cardiac function may experience little or no disability. However, a severe valve deformity may place a serious strain upon the heart, eventually causing heart failure many years after the initial attack of rheumatic fever. When an individual is seriously disabled by a rheumatic valvular deformity, it is possible to excise surgically the abnormal, scarred heart valve and replace it with an artificial valve.

PREVENTION.—Rheumatic heart disease can be largely prevented by the prompt treatment of beta streptococcal infection, thereby forestalling the hypersensitivity state which causes rheumatic fever. Since the person who has once had rheumatic fever is susceptible to recurrent attacks after beta streptococcal infections, many physicians recommend that persons who have had rheumatic fever receive prophylactic penicillin therapy throughout childhood and young adulthood. Penicillin treatment prevents streptococcal infections and reduces the risk of recurrent rheumatic fever and further heart valve damage.

BACTERIAL ENDOCARDITIS

Bacterial endocarditis may be a complication of rheumatic heart disease. A valve damaged by rheumatic fever is susceptible to infection. Small deposits of fibrin may form on the roughened surface of the valve, serving as a site for implantation of bacteria. Transient bacteremias develop occasionally from superficial skin infections, after tooth extractions, and occasionally in association with various minor infections. In a normal person, transient bacteremia causes no problems, since the organisms are rapidly destroyed by the body's normal defenses. However, the individual with a damaged heart valve runs the risk of implanting bacteria on the damaged valve and developing a bacterial inflammation of the heart valve, called *bacterial endocarditis*. Frequently thrombi form at the site of the valve infection, and bits of thrombus may be dislodged and carried as emboli to other parts of the body, producing infarcts in various organs. Because of the hazards of bacterial endocarditis in persons with damaged heart valves, prophylactic antibiotic therapy is commonly given for several days to susceptible individuals about to undergo a tooth extraction or elective surgical procedure. Febrile illnesses in such persons are also treated promptly with appropriate antibiotics. Prophylactic antibiotic therapy given to prevent streptococcal infection in persons who have had rheumatic fever is also effective in preventing the development of bacterial endocarditis.

Coronary Heart Disease

Coronary heart disease results from arteriosclerosis of the large coronary arteries. The arteries narrow due to accumulation of fatty materials within the vessel walls. The lipid deposits, consisting of neutral fat and cholesterol, accumulate in the arteries by diffusion from the bloodstream. Initially, the lipid is contained within mononuclear phagocytic cells in the portion of the artery closest to the lumen. The fatty deposits eventually coalesce, forming pools of fatty material. This is followed by scarring, calcification, and other degenerative changes. The end result is an irregular mass of yellow, mushy debris which encroaches on the lumen of the artery and also extends more deeply into the muscular and elastic tissue of the arterial wall. Often the smooth internal lining of the vessel becomes ulcerated over the surface of the fatty deposits, leaving a roughened surface which predisposes to thrombus formation. The plaque-like deposit of material is called an *atheromatous plaque* or *atheroma* (*athere* = mush); the term for this type of arteriosclerosis is *atherosclerosis*.

CLINICAL FEATURES OF CORONARY HEART DISEASE.—The patient with coronary arteriosclerosis often develops precordial pain on exertion, generally described as *angina pectoris* (pain of the chest). The pain is a result of inadequate blood supply to the heart muscle. It subsides if the patient rests. The lining of the coronary arteries is roughened, and an artery may become completely blocked either by a thrombus or by masses of atherosclerotic debris. This often produces a myocardial infarction in the area of distribution of the blocked vessel. The infarction is associated with severe chest pain and often shock and collapse. Death may occur suddenly after blockage of a large coronary artery, sometimes due to a marked disturbance in cardiac rhythm in which the ventricles fail to contract normally. In other patients, death may be due to rupture of the heart through the area of infarction, leading to leakage of blood into the pericardial sac. Some patients may not have enough surviving heart muscle to maintain normal cardiac function after the infarction and may die of heart failure. If the infarction extends to involve the endocardial lining of the heart, thrombus material may form on the damaged area of endocardium within the left ventricular chamber. Portions of the adherent thrombus material may break loose and form emboli, causing infarctions in spleen, brain, kidney, or other organs. Fortunately, about 80 per cent of patients survive the infarction, and the area of muscle necrosis is replaced by scar tissue.

TREATMENT OF MYOCARDIAL INFARCTION.—Treatment consists of bed rest for several weeks, after which the patient is slowly allowed to resume full activity. Sometimes the injured heart is quite irritable and prone to abnormal rhythms. Therefore, various drugs are often given to decrease the irritability of the heart muscle. The patient who has sustained a myocardial infarction is likely to develop intracardiac thrombi if the endocardium is injured. Or, he may develop thrombi in leg veins due to prolonged bed rest. Therefore, many physicians also administer anticoagulant drugs to reduce the coagulability of the blood and thereby decrease the likelihood of thromboses and emboli. If the patient shows evidence of heart failure, various drugs are administered to sustain the failing heart.

RECENT ADVANCES IN DIAGNOSIS AND TREATMENT OF CORONARY HEART DISEASE.—Physicians can now evaluate the extent of coronary artery disease as well as the exact sites of obstruction of the main coronary arteries. This is accomplished by means of passing a catheter into the aorta and injecting a radiopaque dye directly into the orifices of the coronary arteries. The filling of the coronary arteries can be observed, along with the location and degree of arterial obstruction.

Several surgical approaches have been devised to improve blood supply to the heart muscle. It is sometimes possible to "ream out" the atherosclerotic lining of a narrowed or occluded vessel. This is called *endarterectomy* (*endo* = within + artery). Sometimes a blocked segment of coronary artery can be bypassed by grafting a segment of vein between the aorta and the coronary artery distal to the area of obstruction. A third approach to improve blood flow to the heart muscle is to implant the internal mammary arteries directly into the myocardium. (The internal mammary arteries arise from the aorta and descend along the undersurface of the breast bone.) The transplanted arteries eventually establish contact with the vascular bed of the myocardium and augment the blood supply to the heart muscle.

Blood Lipids and Coronary Artery Disease

The level of lipids in the blood has been shown to be one factor concerned in the pathogenesis of coronary atherosclerosis. The lipids of clinical importance are neutral fat (triglyceride) and cholesterol.

NEUTRAL FAT

Chemically, fat is composed of three molecules of fatty acid combined with one molecule of glycerol. Glycerol is a three-carbon alcohol containing a hydroxyl group (OH) attached to each carbon atom. A fatty acid is a long, straight-chain carbon compound containing a terminal carboxyl group (COOH); this constitutes the acid group of organic molecules. The carboxyl groups of the fatty acids are linked to the hydroxyl groups of glycerol, with loss of a molecule of water, in a linkage called an ester. Neutral fat is frequently referred to as *triglyceride*.

A neutral fat may be classified as saturated or unsaturated. In unsaturated fats, the fatty acids linked to glycerol contain one or more double bonds between adjacent carbon atoms in the molecule. A polyunsaturated fat is one in which the fatty acids contain several double bonds. A saturated fat is one in which there are no double bonds in the fatty acid molecules. At room temperature, saturated fats are solid, whereas unsaturated fats are liquid. In general, fats of animal origin are saturated. Vegetable oils and fats found in fish and poultry are primarily unsaturated.

High levels of neutral fat (along with cholesterol) in the blood promote atherosclerosis. Many investigators believe that elevated triglycerides may be more important than elevated cholesterol in predisposing an individual to atherosclerosis. Carbohydrate is converted readily into fat in the body, and much of the blood triglyceride is derived not from ingested fat but from ingested carbohydrate. In clinical medicine, most examples of high blood triglycerides can be traced to excessively high carbohydrate diets. Sugar has been found to be more potent in elevating blood triglycerides than the more complex carbohydrates derived from cereals and other starches.

Cholesterol

Cholesterol is a complex carbon compound containing several ring structures and is classified as a *sterol*. Most cholesterol is present in the body in combination with fatty acids as cholesterol esters. Cholesterol is synthesized in the body and is also present in many foods. Normally, cholesterol is excreted in the bile into the gastrointestinal tract.

Much evidence indicates that a high dietary intake of cholesterol leads to high levels of blood cholesterol and premature atherosclerosis. Americans subsist on a diet relatively high in cholesterol; they also have one of the highest death rates from coronary heart disease. In contrast, other populations (whose diet is much lower in cholesterol) have a much lower death rate from coronary heart disease.

The level of blood cholesterol is influenced not only by the amount of cholesterol in the diet, but also by the type of dietary fat. Saturated fats, the type found in meats and dairy products, tend to raise blood cholesterol. On the other hand, unsaturated fats, which are found in fish, poultry, and vegetable oils, tend to lower blood cholesterol. The reason for this is unknown. Cholesterol and saturated fat are found together in many foods. In general, foods high in cholesterol also have a high content of saturated fats, whereas foods low in cholesterol contain polyunsaturated fats rather than saturated fats.

ALTERATION OF BLOOD LIPIDS BY CHANGE IN DIET

Various studies have demonstrated that the levels of both cholesterol and triglycerides in the blood can be lowered by dietary change. These studies have also demonstrated that individuals maintained on a modified diet have a lower incidence of coronary artery disease than a comparable group subsisting on an average American diet. The diet (often called an "anticoronary" diet) is modified by decreasing the amount of cholesterol and saturated fat in the diet and substituting foods containing polyunsaturated fats. This involves restricting the intake of animal fat and substituting fish and poultry. Carbohydrates are derived primarily from starches and cereals. The consumption of sugar and foods rich in sugar (pies, cakes, candies, etc.) is reduced, and alcohol consumption is restricted. (Chemically, alcohol is closely related to sugar.)

Modification of the typical American diet is difficult, since it involves breaking old dietary habits. However, some change in diet is desirable since it would significantly reduce the incidence of coronary artery disease in our population. An "anticoronary" diet is essential for individuals who have high levels of blood lipids, since they run a greatly increased risk of death or disability from coronary artery disease.

It should be emphasized that the factors influencing the development of atherosclerosis are complex; an elevated level of blood lipids is only one of many factors concerned with atherogenesis. A number of other conditions, among them obesity, hypertension, cigarette-smoking, and genetic factors, also predispose individuals to atherosclerosis.

Hypertension and Hypertensive Cardiovascular Disease

Hypertension results from excessive vasoconstriction of the small arterioles throughout the body; this, in turn, raises the diastolic blood pressure. Because of the high peripheral resistance, the heart is required to increase the force of ventricular contraction in order to supply blood to the tissues, which produces a compensatory increase in the systolic blood pressure. Marked hypertension exerts injurious effects not only on the heart but on the blood vessels and kidneys.

CARDIAC EFFECTS

The heart responds to the increased work load resulting from the high peripheral resistance by becoming enlarged. Although the enlarged heart may be able to function effectively for many years, the cardiac pump is being forced to work beyond its "rated capacity." Eventually, the heart can no longer maintain adequate blood flow, and the patient develops symptoms of cardiac failure.

Vascular Effects

Because the blood vessels are not designed to carry blood at such a high pressure, the vessels wear out prematurely. Hypertension accelerates the development of atherosclerosis in the larger arteries. The arterioles are also injured; they undergo thickening and degenerative changes, and their lumens become narrowed. This process is termed *arteriolosclerosis*. Sometimes the walls of the small arterioles become completely necrotic due to the effects of the sustained high blood pressure. Weakened arterioles may rupture, leading to hemorrhage. The brain is particularly vulnerable, cerebral hemorrhage being a relatively common complication of marked hypertension.

Renal Effects

The narrowing of the renal arterioles decreases the blood supply to the kidney, which, in turn, leads to injury and degenerative changes in the glomeruli and renal tubules. Severe hypertension may cause marked derangement of renal function and eventually lead to renal failure.

Cause and Treatment of Hypertension

Occasionally, hypertension is due to an adrenal tumor secreting hormones which elevate the blood pressure. Certain uncommon types of renal disease may also occasionally cause hypertension. However, in most instances, the reason for excessive vasoconstriction in the peripheral arterioles is unknown.

Although the reason for the hypertension cannot be determined in most instances, the blood pressure can be reduced to more normal levels, thereby lowering the risk of the various complications of high blood pressure. This is accomplished by administering various drugs which lower the blood pressure by lessening the vasoconstriction of the peripheral blood vessels.

Heart Failure

Heart failure exists whenever the heart is no longer able to pump adequate amounts of blood to the tissues. It may result from any type of

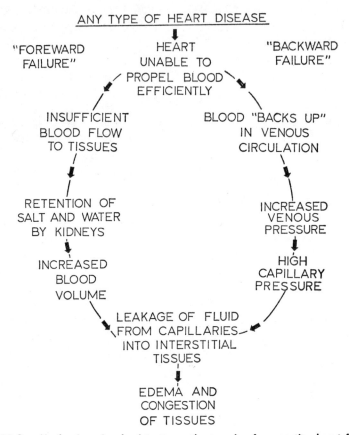

ANY TYPE OF HEART DISEASE

"FOREWARD
FAILURE"

HEART
UNABLE TO
PROPEL BLOOD
EFFICIENTLY

"BACKWARD
FAILURE"

INSUFFICIENT
BLOOD FLOW
TO TISSUES

BLOOD "BACKS UP"
IN VENOUS
CIRCULATION

RETENTION OF
SALT AND WATER
BY KIDNEYS

INCREASED
VENOUS
PRESSURE

INCREASED
BLOOD
VOLUME

HIGH
CAPILLARY
PRESSURE

LEAKAGE OF FLUID
FROM CAPILLARIES
INTO INTERSTITIAL
TISSUES

EDEMA AND
CONGESTION
OF TISSUES

Fig. 15-2.—Mechanisms involved in the pathogenesis of congestive heart failure.

heart disease. Rapid failing of the heart, as when a large portion of muscle undergoes infarction, is called *acute heart failure.* In most cases, however, cardiac failure develops slowly and insidiously; this is called *chronic heart failure.* Since the most prominent feature in chronic heart failure is congestion of the tissues due to engorgement by blood, the physician often uses the term "congestive heart failure" when referring to chronic heart failure and its attendant clinical manifestations.

Sometimes the terms "forward failure" and "backward failure" are used to describe the mechanisms leading to the development of heart failure. In forward failure, the initial effect of inadequate cardiac output is considered to be insufficient blood flow to the tissues. The inadequate renal blood flow results in retention of salt and water by the kidneys. (This effect is mediated indirectly through the adrenal glands.) Fluid retention, in turn, leads to an increased blood volume, and this is soon followed by a rise in venous pressure. The high venous pressure and high capillary pressure cause excessive transudation of fluid from the capillaries, leading to edema of the tissues. In backward failure, the inadequate output of blood is considered to cause "back-up" of blood within the veins draining back to the heart, leading to increased venous pressure, congestion of the viscera, and edema. Figure 15-2 illustrates the interrelationship of the various factors concerned in the development of cardiac failure. Probably both forward failure and backward failure are present to some degree in every patient with heart failure.

Acute Pulmonary Edema

Acute pulmonary edema is a manifestation of acute heart failure. It is caused by a temporary disproportion in the output of blood from the two ventricles. If the output of blood from the left ventricle is temporarily reduced more than the output from the right ventricle, the "right heart" will pump blood into the lungs faster than the "left heart" can deliver the blood to the peripheral tissues. This rapidly engorges the lungs with blood, raises the pulmonary capillary pressure, and produces transudation of fluid into the pulmonary alveoli. The patient becomes extremely short of breath due to accumulation of fluid within the alveoli, and oxygenation of the blood circulating through the lungs is impaired. The edema fluid becomes mixed with inspired air, forming a frothy mixture which "overflows" into the bronchi and trachea, filling the patient's upper respiratory passages.

Aneurysm

An aneurysm is a dilatation of the wall of an artery or an outpouching of a portion of the wall. Most aneurysms are acquired, due to arteriosclerosis which causes weakening of the vessel wall. One type of aneurysm involving the cerebral arteries is due to a congenital abnormality of the vessel wall.

ARTERIOSCLEROTIC ANEURYSM

A small artery which undergoes arteriosclerotic change becomes narrowed and may eventually become thrombosed. A large artery, such as the aorta, has such a large diameter that complete obstruction is uncommon. However, atheromatous deposits tend to damage the wall of the aorta, reducing its elasticity and weakening the wall. The aortic wall tends to balloon out under the stress of the high pressure within the vessel. Aortic aneurysms usually develop in the distal part of the abdominal aorta, since the pressure is highest in this portion of the artery. Aortic aneurysms are dangerous, because they may rupture, leading to massive and often fatal hemorrhage. The treatment of aneurysm is surgical excision of the dilated portion and replacement of the diseased segment by a graft of nylon or Dacron. Occasionally, arteriosclerotic aneurysms develop in other large arteries.

CONGENITAL ANEURYSM

An uncommon type of aneurysm involves the large cerebral arteries at the base of the brain. It is due to a congenital defect in the muscular tissue of the vessel wall, usually at the point where the artery branches. Because of the congenital weakness in the wall, the lining of the arterial wall eventually protrudes through the defect at the point of branching, leading to the formation of a sac-like outpouching.

Although the weakness of the vessel wall is congenital, the actual aneurysm does not develop until many years later, in young adulthood or middle age. These aneurysms are hazardous because they may rupture, producing severe and sometimes fatal hemorrhage within the cranial cavity.

Chapter 16

The Hematopoietic System

Composition and Function of Human Blood

BLOOD IS ESSENTIAL to transport oxygen and nutrients to the tissues, carbon dioxide and other waste products of cell metabolism to the various excretory organs, and leukocytes to various locations in the body. The volume of blood varies with the size of the individual; in the average healthy male, the blood volume is about 5 quarts. Almost half of the blood consists of cellular elements: the red cells, white cells, and platelets.

Red cells, which are concerned primarily with oxygen transport, are the most numerous cells, averaging about five million per cubic millimeter (cu mm) of blood (1 ml = 1,000 cu mm). Red cells normally survive about 4 months in the circulation.

White blood cells are much less numerous, averaging about 7,000 per cubic millimeter. The following cell types are recognized: neutrophils, eosinophils, basophils, monocytes, and lymphocytes. Although lymphocytes are produced chiefly in the lymph nodes and spleen, they are also manufactured in the bone marrow and elsewhere throughout the body where lymphoid tissue is present. Under normal circumstances, production of the other white cells is confined to the bone marrow. In contrast to the relatively long survival of red cells, most white cells have a short survival time within the circulation, varying from several hours to several days, and they must be replenished continually. Lymphocytes are an exception. Two populations of lymphocytes are present in the circulation, one surviving about the same length of time as most of the other leukocytes and another surviving for several years.

The proportions of the various leukocytes vary with the age of the individual. The most numerous white cells in the adult are the neutrophils, constituting about 70 per cent of the total circulating white cells. These are actively phagocytic and are the predominant cells in acute inflammatory reactions. Lymphocytes are the next most frequent type of white cells in the adult and are the predominant leukocytes in the blood of the child. The lymphocytes in the peripheral blood constitute only a small fraction of the total lymphocytes, most being located in the lymph nodes, spleen, and other lymphoid tissues. Lymphocytes continually recirculate from the bloodstream into lymphoid tissues, eventually leaving the lymphoid tissue via lymphatic channels and the thoracic duct, returning to the circulation, and later becoming reestablished for a time in another site of lymphoid tissue. Lymphocytes are concerned with cell-mediated and humoral defense reactions, as has been described.

Small numbers of eosinophils, basophils, and monocytes are also normally present in the blood. Eosinophils are related in some manner to allergy, but their exact function is unknown. Eosinophils increase in allergic diseases and in the presence of worm or other animal parasite infestations. The function of basophils is also unknown. Monocytes are actively phagocytic and increase in certain types of chronic infections. As previously discussed, monocyte-lymphocyte interaction is necessary in the initial phase of response to foreign antigen; it also plays a role in the cell-mediated immune reaction.

Blood platelets, which are essential for normal blood coagulation, are much smaller than leukocytes and represent bits of the cytoplasm of megakaryocytes. The latter are the large precursor cells present in the bone marrow. Platelets have a short survival, comparable to that of most leukocytes.

Normal Hematopoiesis

The bone marrow can be compared to a large manufacturing plant which replenishes the blood cells that are continually being worn out and removed from the circulation. As with any manufacturing process, adequate quantities of raw materials are required. Moreover, the factory must be able to process these raw materials efficiently into finished products (the blood cells). The major raw materials necessary for hematopoiesis are protein, vitamin B_{12}, folic acid (one of the vitamin B group), and iron. Inadequate supplies of these substances will handicap the production of blood cells.

REGULATION OF HEMATOPOIESIS

Red cell production is regulated by the oxygen content of the arterial blood. Decreased oxygen supply to the tissues stimulates erythropoiesis. However, low oxygen tension does not act directly on the bone marrow. The effect is mediated by the kidneys. Certain specialized cells in the kidneys elaborate a hormone-like material which interacts with certain factors in the plasma, leading to the production of an erythrocyte-stimulating material called *erythropoietin*.

The factors regulating the production of white blood cells and their delivery into the circulation are not well understood. Products of cell necrosis may cause an increase in the number of white blood cells in the peripheral blood. Hormone secretion by the adrenals and some other endocrine glands also influences white cell production.

Anemia

Anemia literally means "without blood." Specifically, the term is used to refer to decrease in red cells or subnormal hemoglobin levels. Many classifications of anemia have been proposed, and two different methods of classification are widely used. One system, based on the factor responsible for the anemia, is an etiologic classification. A second system, based on the shape and appearance of the red blood cells (as determined from microscopic examination of a stained blood smear), is a morphologic classification.

ETIOLOGIC CLASSIFICATION OF ANEMIA

One simple classification of the anemias is based on the "bone-marrow-factory" concept (Fig. 16-1). Anemia is classified as due to either inade-

Fig. 16-1.—Classification of anemia based on "bone-marrow-factory" concept.

RAW MATERIALS	FACTORY	FINISHED PRODUCT
PROTEIN VITAMIN B-12 FOLIC ACID IRON		RED CELLS WHITE CELLS PLATELETS
INADEQUATE	PRODUCTION	EXCESSIVE LOSS
INSUFFICIENT RAW MATERIALS	FACTORY DAMAGED	EXTERNAL LOSS HEMOLYSIS

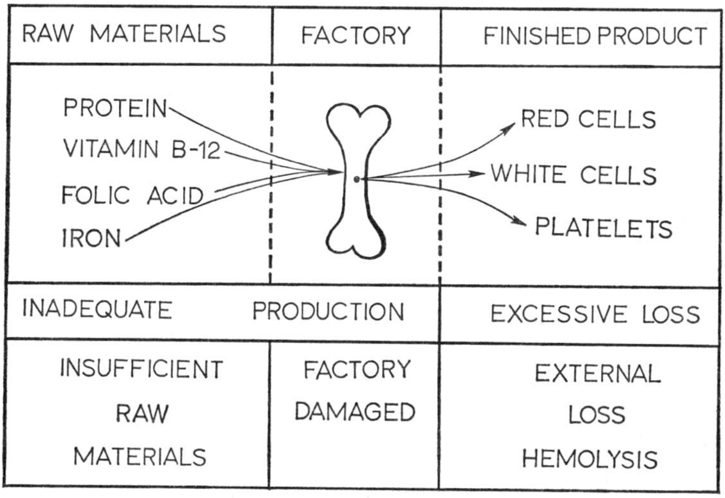

TABLE 16-1.—Etiologic Classification of Anemi

Due to Inadequate Production of Red Cells

1. Inadequate "raw materials"
   A. Iron deficiency anemia
   B. Vitamin B_{12} deficiency
   C. Folic acid deficiency
2. "Bone marrow factory" damaged or inoperative
   A. Marrow depression or destruction (aplastic anemia)
   B. Replacement of marrow by foreign or abnormal cells (myelophthisic anemia)

Due to Excessive Loss of Red Cells

1. External blood loss
2. Shortened survival of red cells in the circulation (hemolytic anemia)
   A. Due to defective red cells (congenital hemolytic anemia)
      Abnormal shape of red cells
      Abnormal hemoglobin in red cells
      Deficient enzymes in red cells
   B. Due to "hostile environment" (acquired hemolytic anemia)
      Due to autoantibodies (autoimmune hemolytic anemia)
      Due to mechanical trauma to red cells

quate production of red cells or excessive loss of cells. Inadequate production, in turn, may result from insufficient raw materials or factors which render the factory inoperative and no longer able to deliver enough finished products into the circulation. Examples of the latter would be marrow damage or replacement of marrow by abnormal cells. Excessive loss of red cells may be due to either external blood loss or accelerated destruction of the cells (and hence shortened survival) in the circulation. Table 16-1 is a tabular classification of the various causes of anemia.

Morphologic Classification of Anemia

An anemia in which the cells are normal in size and appearance is called a *normocytic anemia*. If the cells are larger than normal, the anemia is called a *macrocytic anemia*. If the cells are smaller than normal, the anemia is called a *microcytic anemia*. Many times, microcytic cells also have a reduced hemoglobin content, appearing quite pale when examined under the microscope; here, the term *hypochromic anemia* is used. Often the latter two terms are combined, and the anemia is called a *hypochromic microcytic anemia*. Classification of anemia based on appearance of the red cells is useful, since the appearance of the cells provides a clue to the etiology. Iron-deficiency anemia is a hypochromic microcytic anemia. Anemia due to vitamin B_{12} or folic acid deficiency is a macrocytic anemia. Most other types of anemia are normocytic.

Iron-Deficiency Anemia

Iron-deficiency anemia is the most common anemia encountered in clinical practice. Hemoglobin is an iron-containing protein, and normal synthesis of hemoglobin requires adequate supplies of iron. Iron is absorbed with difficulty from the gastrointestinal tract, and iron stores within the body are carefully conserved. When "senile" red blood cells, which have a normal life span of about 4 months, are removed from the circulation, the iron from the destroyed cells is reused by the bone marrow to be incorporated into newly formed red cells. Iron-deficiency anemia may result from either insufficient intake of iron in the diet or inadequate reutilization of the iron present in red cells.

Iron-deficiency anemia due to inadequate dietary intake is likely to occur in infants and adolescents during periods of rapid growth, when the production of red cells accelerates to supply the needs of an increasing blood volume. During these critical times, if dietary iron is insufficient, the iron supplies for hematopoiesis are inadequate. If an infant is fed only milk (a poor source of iron) and the diet is not supplemented with cereals, fruits, vegetables, and other foods containing iron, iron stores will become rapidly exhausted and iron-deficiency anemia will develop within the first year of life. For this reason, physicians start infants on supplementary foods within the first few months after birth. Occasionally, adolescents subsisting on an inadequate or poorly balanced diet develop an iron-deficiency anemia.

A second common cause of iron-deficiency anemia is failure to recapture the iron present in red cells for hemoglobin synthesis. This is due to chronic blood loss. The iron contained in red cells lost from the circulation by bleeding is no longer available to the body for the production of new red cells. Unless dietary intake of iron is extremely liberal, iron stores soon become exhausted and iron-deficiency anemia develops.

Iron-deficiency anemia is a hypochromic microcytic anemia. The cells are pale because they contain less hemoglobin than normal. The cells are also abnormally small, since the body apparently attempts to "scale down" the size of the cell to conform to the reduced hemoglobin content.

A physician treating a patient with iron-deficiency anemia is primarily concerned with learning the cause of the anemia and then directing therapy toward the cause rather than the symptoms. In an infant with a history of a very poor diet, the cause may be obvious. In an adult, the anemia usually reflects blood loss, and the physician always investigates to determine the source of the bleeding. Blood loss may be due to a bleeding ulcer or an ulcerated carcinoma of the colon. In women, excessive menstrual bleeding is a common cause of iron-deficiency anemia. Once the cause of the blood loss has been determined, proper treatment of the underlying disease can be instituted. In addition, the patient is given supplementary iron to replenish the body's depleted iron stores.

Vitamin B$_{12}$ and Folic Acid Deficiency

Vitamin B$_{12}$ is found in meat, liver, and other foods rich in animal protein. Folic acid is widely distributed in nature, being found in abundance in green leafy vegetables as well as many foods of animal origin.

Vitamin B$_{12}$ and folic acid are required not only for normal hematopoiesis, but for normal maturation of many other types of cells. In the absence of either vitamin B$_{12}$ or folic acid, the developing red cells in the bone marrow exhibit a characteristic disturbance of cell maturation. The developing red cells, which are larger than normal, are called *megaloblasts* (*megalos* = large). The abnormal red cell maturation is called *megaloblastic erythropoiesis*. The mature red cells derived from the abnormal maturation are larger than normal. Therefore, the anemia is classified morphologically as a macrocytic anemia. The development of white cell precursors and megakaryocytes is also abnormal. Consequently, patients with megaloblastic anemia usually also have *leukopenia* and *thrombocytopenia* as well as a macrocytic anemia. Vitamin B$_{12}$, but not folic acid, is required to maintain the structural and functional integrity of the nervous system; thus, a deficiency of this vitamin is often associated with pronounced neurologic disturbances.

Anemia due to folic acid deficiency.—Anemia due to folic acid deficiency is quite uncommon in this country. Occasionally it may be encountered in an individual who has been subsisting on a highly abnormal diet or in a person with a chronic intestinal disease, in whom absorption of folic acid is impaired. Occasionally a megaloblastic anemia due to folic acid deficiency develops in pregnancy. This is due to temporary interference with the metabolism or utilization of folic acid which is related to the pregnancy.

Anemia due to vitamin B$_{12}$ deficiency (pernicious anemia).—Efficient absorption of the vitamin B$_{12}$ ingested in food requires a substance called *intrinsic factor*, secreted by the gastric mucosal cells along with hydrochloric acid and digestive enzymes. Intrinsic factor facilitates the absorption of vitamin B$_{12}$ in the small intestine. The absorbed vitamin is stored in the liver and made available to the bone marrow and other tissues as required for cell growth and maturation.

The basic defect in pernicious anemia is atrophy of the gastric mucosa which sometimes develops in middle-aged and elderly individuals. This results in failure of secretion of intrinsic factor (as well as acid and digestive enzymes), which in turn leads to failure of absorption of vitamin B_{12}. The vitamin B_{12} deficiency causes impaired hematopoiesis as well as various neurologic disturbances.

The treatment of pernicious anemia is intramuscular administration of vitamin B_{12}. Parenteral administration avoids the problem of poor absorption of the vitamin due to lack of intrinsic factor.

BONE MARROW DAMAGE OR INFILTRATION

Hematopoietic cells are relatively sensitive and can be damaged by a large number of injurious substances. Various drugs, chemicals, and exposure to excessive radiation may damage or destroy hematopoietic cells. In some cases, the cause of the marrow injury cannot be determined. This type of anemia, which is due to bone marrow failure, is called *aplastic anemia* (a = without + *plasia* = growth). This term is not strictly accurate, since all hematopoietic precursors are damaged, and leukopenia and thrombocytopenia are present as well as anemia. The red cells in aplastic anemia are normal in size and shape, but inadequate in number. Therefore, aplastic anemia is classified as a normocytic anemia.

A similar type of anemia is produced if marrow cells are crowded out and replaced by abnormal cells, such as leukemic cells or metastatic tumor. As a consequence, there is inadequate production of all blood cells. The anemia is normocytic, and leukopenia and thrombocytopenia also tend to be present. The term *myelophthisic anemia* (*myelo* = marrow + *phthisis* = wasting or decay) is sometimes used to denote any type of anemia caused by infiltration of the bone marrow and consequent displacement of normal marrow cells.

ACUTE BLOOD LOSS OR ACCELERATED BLOOD DESTRUCTION

A normocytic anemia may result from an episode of acute blood loss (for example, a massive hemorrhage from the uterus or gastrointestinal tract). Provided iron stores are adequate, the lost blood is regenerated rapidly by the bone marrow. This is in contrast to the anemia of chronic blood loss, which is a hypochromic microcytic anemia resulting from depletion of iron stores due to prolonged bleeding.

HEMOLYTIC ANEMIA.—Normally, red cells survive about 4 months. Sometimes the survival of red cells in the circulation is markedly shortened, and anemia develops because the regenerative capacity of the marrow is unable to keep up with the accelerated destruction. *Hemolytic anemia* may be due to defective red cells (congenital hemolytic anemia) or a "hostile environment" (acquired hemolytic anemia).

Congenital hemolytic anemia.—Some individuals have genetically determined abnormalities of their red cells, so that the cells are unable to survive normally in the circulation. The congenital defect may manifest itself in the production of abnormally shaped cells, cells containing an abnormal hemoglobin, or cells deficient in enzymes necessary for normal cell survival.

Normally, the red cell is a circular, biconcave disk. Some hereditary conditions are characterized by the formation of cells which are more spherical than normal (hereditary spherocytosis) or oval rather than circular (ovalocytosis).

The hemoglobin within the cell may be abnormal, often leading to a shortened red cell survival. Many different kinds of abnormal hemoglobin have been described. Hemoglobin S (sickle cell hemoglobin) is one of the more common. Sickle cell hemoglobin is common among Negroes and may be associated with a hemolytic anemia under certain conditions. The hemoglobin is insoluble under reduced oxygen tension and crystallizes out of solution within the red cells, leading to distortion of the cells.

Red cells derive energy from breakdown of glucose by complex enzymatic reactions. Some individuals have genetically determined deficiencies of enzymes that are necessary for normal metabolic functions of the red cells. Such enzyme-deficient cells are highly susceptible to injury from various causes and cannot survive normally. A large number of genetically determined enzyme deficiencies have been identified which can lead to premature destruction of red cells under certain conditions.

Acquired hemolytic anemia.—Sometimes the red cells are normally formed but incapable of normal survival because the cells are injured in the circulation. The cells have been released into a "hostile environment." For example, some patients develop autoantibodies directed against their own red cells, leading to accelerated destruction of the cells. Some of the collagen diseases and some diseases of the lymphatic system are associated with hemolytic anemia due to autoantibodies. This type of hemolytic anemia is often termed *autoimmune hemolytic anemia.*

In another type of acquired hemolytic anemia, red cells may be destroyed by mechanical trauma. Some diseases are characterized by marked enlargement of the spleen. Red cells passing through a very large spleen may be subject to considerable mechanical trauma, accelerating their destruction. Occasionally, a hemolytic anemia may follow the insertion of an artificial heart valve. The red cells are injured by contact against some part of the artificial valve.

Evaluation of Anemia by the Physician

When a patient presents with an anemia, the physician's function is to determine the cause so that proper, effective treatment can be instituted. A careful medical history and physical examination may provide important clues to the most likely cause. A complete blood count is essential in order to assess the degree of anemia and to determine whether leukopenia and thrombocytopenia are also present. Careful microscopic examination of a blood smear allows the physician to determine whether the anemia is hypochromic microcytic, normocytic, or macrocytic; this information is helpful in identifying the probable cause of the anemia. The rate of production of new red cells can be determined by a *reticulocyte count*. Young, newly produced red cells are called *reticulocytes* and can be distinguished by special staining procedures. An elevated reticulocyte count suggests rapid regeneration of red cells, as would be seen after acute blood loss or hemolysis. Many times, a bone marrow examination is also desirable. In this procedure, a small amount of bone marrow is aspirated from the sternum or other site and examined microscopically. Characteristic abnormalities in the maturation of the marrow cells are seen in pernicious anemia and in anemia due to folic acid deficiency. Bone marrow examination also detects interference with bone marrow functions secondary to infiltration by leukemic cells or metastatic tumor. Aplastic anemia can generally be recognized by bone marrow study. Certain other tests are used when chronic blood loss from the gastrointestinal tract is suspected. Stools are examined for blood, and x-ray studies of the gastrointestinal tract are frequently performed in an attempt to localize a site of bleeding. Various other diagnostic procedures are performed in special circumstances.

Polycythemia

An increase of red cells and hemoglobin above normal levels is called *polycythemia*. Polycythemia may occur secondary to an underlying disease which produces decreased arterial oxygen saturation (secondary polycythemia). Or, it may represent a manifestation of a leukemia-like overproduction of red cells for no apparent reason (primary polycythemia).

Secondary Polycythemia

Any condition associated with decreased arterial oxygen tension leads to increased erythropoietin production and hence increased levels of red cells. This may be due to pulmonary emphysema, pulmonary fibrosis, or other type of chronic lung disease which lowers the oxygenation of the blood. Some types of congenital heart disease associated with shunting of unsaturated venous blood into the systemic circulation lead to low arterial oxygen tension and may cause secondary polycythemia.

Rarely, polycythemia may be due to a renal tumor. Apparently the polycythemia is caused by excess erythropoietin production by the tumor; it subsides after removal of the neoplasm.

PRIMARY POLYCYTHEMIA

This disease, also called *polycythemia vera* ("true polycythemia") is a manifestation of a diffuse hyperplasia of the bone marrow of unknown etiology. It is characterized by overproduction not only of red cells but of white blood cells and platelets. The disease has many features of a neoplastic process, and some patients with polycythemia vera eventually develop granulocytic leukemia.

COMPLICATIONS AND TREATMENT OF POLYCYTHEMIA

The symptoms of polycythemia are related to the increased blood volume and increased blood viscosity. Many patients with polycythemia develop thromboses due to the increased blood viscosity and elevated platelet levels. Polycythemia vera is usually treated by various drugs which suppress the bone marrow overactivity. Secondary polycythemia is sometimes treated by periodic removal of excess blood (phlebotomy).

Thrombocytopenia

Blood platelets are derived from megakaryocytes. The platelets, which are fragments of the cytoplasm of megakaryocytes, are released into the bloodstream. These small structures exert a hemostatic function, sealing small breaks in capillaries and also interacting with plasma factors in the initial stages of blood clotting. A marked reduction in the numbers of platelets in the blood leads to numerous small, pinpoint hemorrhages from capillaries in the skin and mucous membranes and also larger patches of extravasated blood. This latter type of cutaneous hemorrhage is called *purpura,* and the entity is called *thrombocytopenic purpura.* The number of platelets may be reduced by bone marrow disease which impairs platelet production or by accelerated destruction of platelets in the circulation.

Many cases of thrombocytopenic purpura result from damage to the bone marrow by drugs, chemicals, or other substances. Others are due to infiltration of the bone marrow by leukemic cells or metastatic carcinoma. This is called *secondary thrombocytopenic purpura*, since the purpura is the result of an underlying disease of the bone marrow.

Sometimes the production of platelets by the bone marrow is normal, but the platelets are rapidly destroyed in the circulation. Often autoantibodies directed against platelets can be detected in the blood of affected individuals. Cases of this type, in which no underlying disease can be detected, are called *primary thrombocytopenic purpura.* This type of thrombocytopenic purpura is often encountered in children and subsides spontaneously within a short time. When the disease occurs in adults, it tends to be more chronic.

Chapter 17

The Lymphatic System

THE LYMPHATIC SYSTEM consists of the lymph nodes and spleen, together with various organized masses of lymphoid tissue elsewhere throughout the body; these include the tonsils, adenoids, and lymphoid aggregates in the intestinal mucosa and the bone marrow. The lymph nodes, which comprise a major part of the system, form an interconnected network linked by lymphatic channels. The lymph nodes consist of masses of lymphocytes supported by a framework of reticulum cells and fibers. The reticulum cells are phagocytic cells, which are part of the reticuloendothelial system. Lymph nodes have been compared to filters which trap and destroy foreign material draining into the nodes via the lymphatic channels.

The lymphatic system is concerned primarily with the immunologic defenses against foreign material, by means of cell-mediated and humoral defense mechanisms (described previously). The common diseases affecting the lymphatic system are infections and neoplasms.

Inflammation of Lymph Nodes (Lymphadenitis)

Lymph nodes draining an area of infection may become enlarged and tender, due to spread of infection through the lymphatic channels and acute inflammation in the node. This is called *lymphadenitis.*

Infectious Mononucleosis

Infectious mononucleosis, a relatively common viral disease, belongs to the same family as the herpes virus which causes fever blisters. The virus has been named the *Epstein-Barr virus* (usually simply called the "EB virus"). The disease is encountered most frequently in young adults and is transmitted by close contact, often by kissing. The virus causes an acute, debilitating, febrile illness associated with a diffuse hyperplasia of lymphoid tissue throughout the body. The lymphoid hyperplasia is manifested clinically by enlargement and tenderness of lymph nodes, some degree of splenic enlargement, and a moderate increase of lymphocytes in the peripheral blood. The lymphocytes show rather distinctive morphologic abnormalities, and the diagnosis can generally be made by the pathologist from a careful examination of the blood smear. Enlargement and ulceration of lymphoid tissue in the throat is responsible for the sore throat often accompanying the disease.

The blood of patients with infectious mononucleosis frequently contains antibodies capable of clumping sheep red cells. These are called *heterophile antibodies*. Antibodies against the EB virus can also be detected in the blood of most patients. The diagnosis of infectious mononucleosis can be established on the basis of the clinical features of a febrile illness in a young adult with lymphadenopathy, the characteristic appearance of the blood smear, and the presence of heterophile and EB virus antibodies in the patient's blood. The disease is self-limited, and no specific treatment is available.

Neoplasms Involving Lymph Nodes

METASTATIC TUMORS

Lymph nodes may be involved by spread of metastatic tumor from malignant tumors arising in breast, lung, colon, or other sites. The nodes involved first lie in the immediate drainage area of the tumor. The tumor may then spread to other, more distant lymph nodes via lymphatic channels and eventually may gain access to the circulatory system through the thoracic duct.

MALIGNANT LYMPHOMA

A lymphoma is a primary malignant neoplasm of lymphoid tissue. There are three major types of lymphoma: reticulum cell sarcoma, lymphosarcoma, and Hodgkin's disease (described in the section on neoplasms). A lymphoma usually begins in a single lymph node or small group of nodes, but often spreads to other nodes; frequently the disease becomes widespread. The spread of lymphoma to multiple groups of nodes is probably a consequence of the recirculation of lymphocytes within the lymphatic system, as previously described in Chapter 16.

LYMPHOCYTIC LEUKEMIA

Leukemia may develop from lymphoid cells in the bone marrow or from lymphoid tissue elsewhere in the body. Leukemia has been discussed in the section on neoplasms.

Alteration of Immune Reactions in Disease of the Lymphatic System

Because of the central role of the lymphatic system in immune reactions, many diseases involving the lymphatic system diffusely, such as leukemias and lymphomas, are frequently associated with abnormal immune responses. This may be manifested either by production of autoantibodies directed against the red cells, white cells, or platelets of the affected individual, or by loss of normal cell-mediated and humoral defenses, leading to an increased susceptibility to infection.

The Problem of the Enlarged Lymph Node

The patient who visits a physician because one or more lymph nodes are enlarged may present a difficult diagnostic problem. Lymph node enlargement may be a manifestation of a localized infection in the area of drainage of the node, it may be due to a systemic infection with initial manifestations in the node, it may be due to metastatic tumor in the node, or it may be an early manifestation of either leukemia or malignant lymphoma. Often the cause of the lymphadenopathy can be determined by the physician from the clinical evaluation of the patient in conjunction with various laboratory studies, including an examination of the peripheral blood. However, sometimes the cause cannot be established, and the physician must perform a lymph node biopsy to determine the reason for the enlargement. The enlarged lymph node is surgically excised and submitted to the pathologist for microscopic examination and microbiologic studies. Generally, the pathologist can make a specific diagnosis on the basis of these studies.

Chapter 18

The Respiratory System

NORMAL LIFE PROCESSES require the delivery of an adequate supply of oxygen to the tissue and removal of the waste products of cell metabolism. This requires a cooperative effort on the part of both the respiratory and circulatory systems. The respiratory system is concerned with the oxygenation of the blood and the removal of carbon dioxide. The circulatory system (described earlier) is concerned with the transport of these gases in the bloodstream.

Lung Structure and Function

The lungs consist of two separate components. The first is a system of tubes, the bronchi and bronchioles, which carry air in and out of the lungs. The second component is the pulmonary alveoli, where actual gas exchange takes place. Just as a tree branches progressively and eventually ends in a foliage of leaves, so the bronchi branch repeatedly and terminate in clusters of pulmonary alveoli. Each alveolus is surrounded by a rich network of pulmonary capillaries. The blood within the pulmonary capillaries is in intimate contact with the air within the alveoli, being separated only by a thin alveolar lining membrane.

Respiration may be considered to consist of two parts, corresponding to the two structural components of the lungs. The first is *ventilation,* which is concerned with the movement of air in and out of the lungs. The second is *gas exchange* between alveolar air and pulmonary capillaries. Normal ventilation and normal gas exchange are both required for effective respiration.

VENTILATION

Air moves in and out of the lungs as a result of the bellows action of the thoracic cage. During inspiration, the ribs become more horizontal, due to the action of the intercostal muscles, and the diaphragm descends.

Consequently, the volume of the thoracic cage increases. The lungs expand to fill the increased volume of the intrathoracic space, and air is drawn into the lungs through the trachea and bronchi. During expiration, the ribs become more vertical and the diaphragm is elevated. The volume of the thoracic cage is reduced. The lungs, which conform to the size of the thorax, also decrease in volume, and air is expelled.

Normal respiratory movements require normal respiratory muscles, normal innervation of the muscles, and normal mobility of the thoracic cage. Ventilation is impaired if the nerve supply to the respiratory muscles is damaged by disease, such as poliomyelitis, or if the respiratory muscles undergo atrophy and degeneration, as in some uncommon types of muscle disease. Ventilation is also impaired if the thoracic cage is immobile. For example, a person buried in sand up to his neck will suffocate because he is unable to move his thoracic cage and therefore cannot move air in and out of his lungs.

GAS EXCHANGE

Exchange of gases between alveolar air and pulmonary capillaries is accomplished by means of diffusion across the alveolar membrane. Efficient gas exchange requires a large capillary surface area in contact with alveolar air, unimpeded diffusion of gases across the alveolar membrane, normal pulmonary blood flow, and normal pulmonary alveoli.

Exchange of oxygen and carbon dioxide by diffusion is governed by differences in the concentrations (partial pressures) of the gases in the blood and alveolar air. Oxygen diffuses into the blood because the partial pressure of the gas is higher in the alveolar air than in the capillary blood. Carbon dioxide diffuses in the opposite direction because the concentration of carbon dioxide is higher in the pulmonary capillaries than in the alveoli. The spongy structure of the lungs, in which each tiny air sac is surrounded by a large network of capillaries, provides the large surface area required for efficient gas exchange (Fig. 18-1, A). Destruction of alveolar septa leads to coalescence of alveoli and reduction in size of the capillary network surrounding the alveoli, resulting in less efficient gas exchange (Fig. 18-1, B).

If the alveolar septa are thickened and scarred, the free diffusion of gases across the thickened alveolar membranes is impeded (Fig. 18-1, C). Gas exchange is also impaired if pulmonary blood flow is obstructed to a portion of the lung, as might be caused by a pulmonary embolus obstructing a large pulmonary artery or by blockage of pulmonary capillaries by fat emboli or foreign material (Fig. 18-1, D). If the pulmonary alveoli

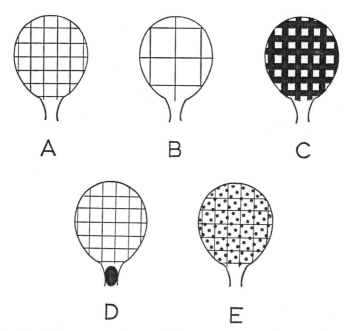

Fig. 18-1.—Various types of structural and functional abnormalities which adversely affect pulmonary gas exchange, as described in text. **A,** normal alveoli and pulmonary blood flow; **B,** destruction of alveolar septa leading to coarsening of alveolar structure with corresponding reduction in the size of the pulmonary capillary bed; **C,** fibrous thickening and scarring of alveolar septa, impeding diffusion of gases across alveolar membrane; **D,** obstruction of pulmonary blood flow to a portion of lung; **E,** alveoli filled with fluid or inflammatory exudate.

become filled with fluid or inflammatory exudate, inspired air cannot enter the diseased alveoli, and pulmonary gas exchange is impeded (Fig. 18-1, *E*).

THE PLEURAL CAVITY

The lungs are covered by a thin membrane called the *pleura*, which is also reflected over the internal surface of the chest wall. Since the lungs fill the thoracic cavity, the two pleural surfaces are in contact. The potential space between the lung and chest wall is the pleural cavity. Normally the apposing pleural surfaces move smoothly over one another. However, in disease the pleural surfaces may become roughened due to inflammation and may become adherent. Inflammatory exudate may accumulate in the pleural cavity and separate the two pleural surfaces.

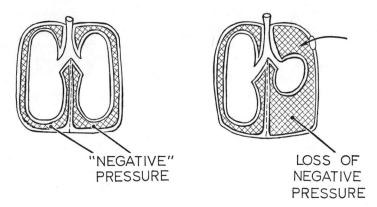

"NEGATIVE" PRESSURE

LOSS OF NEGATIVE PRESSURE

Fig. 18-2.—Left, normal relationship of lung to chest wall. The size of the pleural space is exaggerated. Pleural surfaces are normally in contact. "Negative pressure" is due to tendency of stretched lung to pull away from chest wall. Right, pneumothorax due to perforating injury of chest wall.

INTRAPLEURAL AND INTRAPULMONARY PRESSURES

The lungs are held in an expanded position within the thoracic cavity because the intrapleural pressure is less than the intrapulmonary pressure. The pressure differences are a consequence of the postnatal expansion of the thoracic cavity. The lungs, filled with air at atmospheric pressure, expand to fill the enlarged thoracic cavity, stretching the elastic tissue within the lung. The tendency of the stretched lung to pull away from the chest wall and return to its original contracted state creates the subatmospheric pressure, often called the "negative pressure."

Because of these pressure differences, if a hole is created in the chest wall or in the lung, air at atmospheric pressure enters the pleural space. The negative pressure within the pleural cavity is then abolished, and the stretched lung collapses due to the contraction of the elastic tissue within the lung. This condition is called a *pneumothorax*. A pneumothorax may follow any lung injury or pulmonary disease which permits leakage of air from the lung into the pleural space, or it may follow a perforating injury to the chest wall which allows entry of air at atmospheric pressure into the pleural space (Fig. 18-2).

Pneumonia

Pneumonia is an inflammation of the lung cnaracterized by the same type of vascular changes and exudation of fluid and cells as inflammation in any other location. However, the inflammatory process is influenced by the spongy character of the lungs. The inflammatory exudate spreads unimpeded through the lung, filling the alveoli, and the involved portions of lung become relatively solid (termed *consolidation*). The inflammatory exudate may reach the pleural surface in some areas, causing irritation and inflammation of the pleura; sometimes inflammatory exudate accumulates in the pleural space.

Classification of Pneumonia

Pneumonia may be classified in several ways: by etiology, by anatomic distribution of the inflammatory process, or by predisposing factors which led to its development.

The etiologic classification is the most important, since it serves as a guide to treatment. Pneumonia may be due to bacteria, viruses, or fungi. Whenever possible, the pneumonia is classified in greater detail by designating the exact organism responsible for the disease, such as the pneumococcus or staphylococcus.

The anatomic classification describes whether an entire lobe of the lung is involved, called *lobar pneumonia,* or whether the inflammation involves only portions of one or more lobes immediately adjacent to the bronchi, called *bronchopneumonia.*

Classification of pneumonia by predisposing factors is also common. Any condition associated with poor lung ventilation and retention of bronchial secretions predisposes an individual to the development of pneumonia. Postoperative pneumonia is a pulmonary inflammation which develops in the postsurgical patient who is unable to cough or breathe deeply because of pain; the resultant poor ventilation and retention of secretions lead to pneumonia. Aspiration pneumonia is the result of aspiration of a foreign body, food, vomit, or other irritating substance into the lung. Obstructive pneumonia develops in the lung distal to an area of narrowing or obstruction of a bronchus. Blockage of a bronchus by a tumor or foreign body leads to poor aeration and retention of bronchial secretions in the obstructed portion of lung.

Clinical Features

The signs and symptoms of pneumonia are those of any systemic infection. The patient is ill and has a fever, and the number of white blood cells in the peripheral blood is frequently increased. Bronchial inflammation is evident, manifested by cough and purulent sputum. If the inflammatory process involves the pleura, the patient experiences pain on respiration due to rubbing of the inflamed pleural surfaces against each other. The patient may also have symptoms related to partial loss of lung function. This is due to consolidation of part of the lung secondary to the accumulation of inflammatory cells within the alveoli. Oxygenation of the blood is impaired and the patient may become quite short of breath.

Treatment of pneumonia consists of correcting any predisposing factors which contributed to the development of the pulmonary infection together with appropriate antibiotic therapy.

Tuberculosis

Pulmonary tuberculosis is a special type of pneumonia due to an acid-fast bacterium, the tubercle bacillus (*Mycobacterium tuberculosis*). The tubercle bacillus has a capsule composed of waxes and fatty substances which makes it more resistant to destruction than many other organisms. The body's response to the tubercle bacillus also differs from the usual acute inflammatory reaction; it consists of accumulation of monocytes around the bacteria. Many of the monocytes fuse together, forming rather characteristic large multinucleated cells called "giant cells." Lymphocytes and plasma cells also accumulate, and fibrous tissue proliferates around the central cluster of monocytes and giant cells. Usually the central portion of the cellular aggregation becomes necrotic. This characteristic nodular mass of cells with central necrosis is called a *granuloma,* and the inflammatory process is called a *granulomatous inflammation.*

Course of a Tuberculous Infection

When tubercle bacilli are introduced into the lungs, the typical granulomatous reaction follows. When the number of organisms is small and the body's resistance is high, the inflammation heals by scarring. If a large number of organisms is inhaled, or if the body's defenses are inadequate, the inflammation will progress, causing more marked destruction of lung tissue. Often the granulomatous inflammatory process makes contact with a bronchus, and necrotic inflammatory tissue is discharged into the bronchus. A cavity then forms within the lung, surrounded by granulomatous inflammatory tissue containing masses of tubercle bacilli. The person who has active progressive tuberculosis with a tuberculous cavity can infect others because he is discharging large numbers of tubercle bacilli in his sputum (Fig. 18-3).

In a tuberculous infection of the lung, organisms are often carried in lymphatic channels from the lung into the peribronchial lymph nodes, leading to a tuberculous inflammation in the regional lymph nodes.

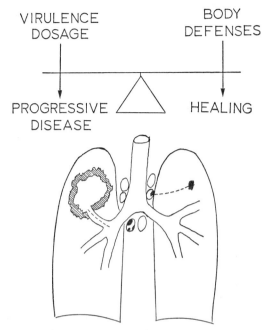

Fig. 18-3.—Possible outcome of a tuberculous inflammation of lung in relation to virulence and dosage of the organism and resistance of the body. The frequent involvement of the regional lymph nodes is indicated. **Left,** progressive disease with cavitation, due to infection with large numbers of organisms or inadequate defenses. **Right,** healing with scarring, due to small numbers of organisms or high degree of resistance to infection.

MILIARY TUBERCULOSIS AND TUBERCULOUS PNEUMONIA

Miliary tuberculosis and tuberculous pneumonia are two uncommon but extremely serious forms of tuberculosis. Miliary tuberculosis develops if a mass of tuberculous inflammatory tissue erodes into a large blood vessel, disseminating large numbers of organisms throughout the body via the bloodstream. The term "miliary" is derived from the resemblance of the multiple foci of disseminated tuberculosis (present in liver, spleen, kidney, and other tissues) to millet seeds. These foci are small white nodules about 1 to 2 mm in diameter. Tuberculous pneumonia is an overwhelming infection characterized by extensive tuberculous consolidation of one or more lobes of the lung.

EXTRAPULMONARY TUBERCULOSIS

Sometimes tuberculosis occurs in kidney, bone, uterus, fallopian tube, or other extrapulmonary location. The infection results from hematogenous spread of tubercle bacilli from a focus of tuberculosis in the lung. Sometimes the pulmonary infection heals, but the secondary focus of infection may progress, leading to an active, extrapulmonary, tuberculous infection without clinically apparent pulmonary tuberculosis.

Diagnosis and Treatment of Tuberculosis

Tuberculous infection is associated with the development of hypersensitivity to proteins in the tubercle bacillus (see Chapter 3). A positive skin test (Mantoux test) indicates that the person was at one time infected with the tubercle bacillus; it does not necessarily indicate an active tuberculous infection.

Tuberculosis is treated by a number of different antibiotics and chemotherapeutic agents. Sometimes surgical resection of diseased lung tissue is also performed. At present, many physicians recommend that persons who develop an infection with the tubercle bacillus, as manifested by conversion from a negative to a positive skin test reaction, be treated with an antituberculosis drug. Treatment is also recommended for patients with inactive tuberculosis who have an increased risk of developing a reactivation of an old, apparently healed tuberculous infection.

It is now well known that old tuberculous lesions which appear completely healed may harbor tubercle bacilli. If the resistance of the patient is lowered by a debilitating disease, treatment with adrenal corticosteroids, or other factors, an apparently healed focus of tuberculosis may flare up, leading to active, progressive tuberculosis. Many cases of active tuberculosis in older patients represent a reactivation of an old infection rather than a new infection by the tubercle bacillus.

Bronchitis and Bronchiectasis

Acute inflammation of the tracheobronchial mucosa is common in many upper respiratory infections. The raw throat and cough associated with many respiratory infections is due to the associated acute bronchitis. Chronic bronchitis is also common; often it results from chronic irritation of the respiratory mucosa by cigarette-smoking or breathing air containing large amounts of atmospheric pollutants.

Sometimes the bronchial walls in parts of the lung become weakened as a result of severe inflammation or other factors, and the involved bronchi become markedly dilated. This condition is called *bronchiectasis* (*ectasia* = dilatation). The distended bronchi tend to retain secretions. Consequently, patients with bronchiectasis frequently have a chronic cough associated with production of large amounts of purulent sputum. Often they suffer repeated bouts of pulmonary infection. The only effective treatment of bronchiectasis is surgical resection of the involved segments of lung. Bronchiectasis can be recognized by means of a special type of radiologic examination called a *bronchogram*. The procedure consists of taking x-ray films after instillation of a radiopaque oil into the trachea and bronchi. The oil covers the mucosa of the bronchi, and the abnormal bronchi can be recognized as dilated saccular or fusiform structures.

Pulmonary Emphysema

Twenty years ago, emphysema was relatively uncommon. Now the disease is an important cause of disability and death, and its incidence is increasing at an alarming rate. In emphysema, the normal fine alveolar structure of the lung is lost because of rupture of alveolar septa, leading to coalescence of alveoli into large, cystic air spaces. As previously described, effective gas exchange between blood and alveolar air requires a large capillary surface area. Progressive destruction of the alveolar septa gradually reduces the size of the capillary bed available for gas exchange.

The chief symptom of emphysema is shortness of breath. Initially this is noted only on exertion, but later may be present even at rest. The patient also usually has a chronic cough with purulent sputum, due to the associated chronic bronchitis. Eventually, the severely affected patient may die because he lacks enough functionally normal lung tissue to sustain life or because of a superimposed pulmonary infection. Emphysema is also a frequent cause of respiratory acidosis, one of the common disturbances of acid-base balance. This will be discussed in Chapter 27.

Pathogenesis of Emphysema

Cigarette-smoking and atmospheric air pollution appear to be the major factors responsible for the rising incidence of emphysema. Exactly how they exert their destructive effect on the lung is not completely understood. Figure 18-4 summarizes one concept of the pathogenesis of this serious and disabling disease. Smoking and air pollution are considered to expose the bronchial mucosa to chronic irritation, eventually producing chronic bronchitis. This is associated with a chronic cough and increased bronchial secretions. The smaller bronchioles become narrowed because of the inflammatory swelling of the mucosa. Consequently, the resistance to expiration increases through the narrowed bronchioles, resulting in trapping of air within the lung. Repeated bouts of coughing, with conse-

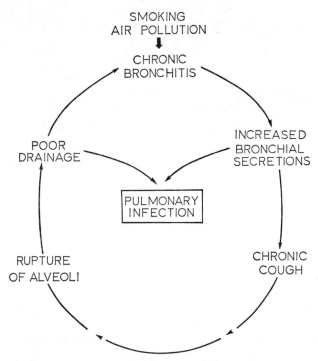

Fig. 18-4.—A concept of the pathogenesis of pulmonary emphysema.

quent marked elevations in intrabronchial pressure, cause rupture of alveolar septa, with gradual conversion of alveoli into large, cystic air spaces. The lungs become overdistended and lose their normal elasticity. The patient cannot expel air normally from the overdistended lungs because of loss of normal lung elasticity and bronchiolar obstruction; he also has difficulty expectorating the excessive bronchial secretions. Retention of secretions and poor drainage of secretions from the bronchi tends to perpetuate the chronic bronchitis, and a vicious circle is created. The diseased lungs are also more susceptible to infection because of impaired pulmonary ventilation, bronchial inflammation, bronchiolar obstruction, and excessive bronchial secretions. Therefore, patients with emphysema frequently have repeated bouts of pneumonia, further damaging the lung tissue.

PREVENTION AND TREATMENT OF EMPHYSEMA

Emphysema can be largely prevented by refraining from smoking and avoiding inhalation of other substances known to be injurious to the lungs.

Atmospheric air pollution contributes to the increasing incidence of emphysema, and various measures are being undertaken to control this serious public health problem.

Once emphysema has developed, the damaged lungs cannot be restored to normal. However, several measures can be employed to promote the drainage of bronchial secretions, to improve pulmonary ventilation, and to decrease the frequency of superimposed pulmonary infections. These measures, along with cessation of smoking, will retard or arrest further progression of the disease.

Pulmonary Fibrosis

The lungs are continually exposed to a number of injurious substances. These consist of various irritant gases discharged into the atmosphere and many kinds of airborne organic and inorganic particles. Severe pulmonary injury may lead to *pulmonary fibrosis*. Fibrous thickening of alveolar septa makes the lungs increasingly rigid, restricting normal respiratory excursions. Diffusion of oxygen and carbon dioxide between alveolar air and pulmonary capillaries is also hampered because of the increased thickness of the alveolar septa (Fig. 18-1, *C*). Pulmonary fibrosis causes progressive respiratory disability similar to that encountered in pulmonary emphysema.

Some types of collagen diseases, characterized by injury to connective tissue, may have as their major manifestation injury to the connective tissue framework of the lung, leading to pulmonary fibrosis.

Certain occupational diseases are recognized as being due to inhalation of injurious substances. The general term *pneumoconiosis* (*pneumo* = lung + *konis* = dust + *osis* = condition) is used to refer to lung injury produced by inhalation of injurious dust or other particulate material. The best-known of the pneumoconioses is *silicosis,* a type of progressive, nodular, pulmonary fibrosis due to inhalation of rock dust. Inhalation of asbestos fibers, cotton fibers, certain types of fungus spores, and many other substances attending certain occupations may also cause pulmonary fibrosis.

Lung Carcinoma

Lung carcinoma is another important disease related to cigarette-smoking. Formerly, lung carcinoma was uncommon. Now this is the most common malignant tumor in men, and the incidence in women is also increasing. The tumor is quite rare in nonsmokers. Since the neoplasm usually arises from the bronchial mucosa, the term *bronchogenic carci-*

noma is often used when referring to lung cancer. Because of the rich lymphatic and vascular network in the lung, the neoplasm readily gains access to lymphatic channels and pulmonary blood vessels and soon spreads to regional lymph nodes and distant sites. Treatment usually consists of surgical resection of one or more lobes of the lung. Radiation therapy rather than surgery is used to treat some types of lung cancer and is also used to treat tumors which are too far advanced for surgical resection. Results of treatment are disappointing because the disease is often widespread by the time it is recognized. This tumor could largely be prevented by elimination of cigarette-smoking.

Chapter 19

The Breast

THE FEMALE BREAST is composed of lobules consisting of glands and branching ducts in fibrofatty tissue. Before puberty, breast tissue consists only of branching ducts and fibrous tissue without glandular tissue or fat. Postpubertal changes involve proliferation of glandular tissue and accumulation of adipose tissue within the breast. Variations in the size of the postpubertal breast of nonpregnant women are due primarily to variations in the amount of fat in the breast rather than differences in the amount of glandular tissue. Mild cyclic hyperplasia followed by involution of breast tissue occurs normally during the menstrual cycle. The glandular and ductal tissues of the breast become markedly hypertrophic under the hormonal stimulus of pregnancy and lactation, and the breast undergoes regression in the postpartum period.

The three common diseases of the breast are benign cystic disease, fibroadenoma, and carcinoma.

Benign Cystic Disease

Benign cystic disease is characterized by focal areas of proliferation of glandular and fibrous tissue in the breast associated with localized dilatation of ducts, resulting in the formation of various-sized cysts in the breast. Cystic disease appears to be due to irregularities in the response of the breast to the normal cyclic variations of each menstrual cycle. Clinically, cystic disease may be manifested as an apparently solitary mass within the breast. Under these circumstances, the lesion is treated by surgical excision since it cannot be distinguished clinically from a neoplasm.

Fibroadenoma

Fibroadenoma is a benign, well-circumscribed tumor of fibrous and glandular breast tissues which is seen most commonly in young women. It is readily cured by simple surgical excision.

Carcinoma

This is the most common malignant tumor in women. It spreads by infiltration and eventually metastasizes to regional lymph nodes and distant sites. Treatment usually consists of radical surgical removal of the breast, pectoral muscles, and axillary tissues. In patients with widespread disease, a number of other measures can be used to produce temporary arrest or regression of the tumor. These include radiation therapy, removal of the ovaries, or administration of certain sex hormones.

The Problem of a Lump in the Breast

Many times the physician is faced with the difficult problem presented by the patient who has a lump in her breast. It may have been detected by the patient herself or by the physician in the course of a routine physical examination. The lump could be benign fibrocystic disease, a benign fibroadenoma, a carcinoma, or one of many other less common diseases of the breast. Certain clinical features may suggest to the physician the probability that the given breast lesion is benign or malignant. However, the only way to be certain is to perform a surgical excision of the mass. This can be examined by the pathologist, who can make an exact diagnosis. If the lesion is benign, no further treatment is necessary. If the lesion proves to be malignant, the surgeon can immediately perform a more extensive surgical operation.

Chapter 20

Diseases of the Female Reproductive System

Gonorrhea

GONORRHEA IS CAUSED by the gonococcus (*Neisseria gonorrhoeae*) and is transmitted by sexual contact. In the female, the gonococcus causes inflammation of the uterine cervix, the urethra and periurethral glands, and often Bartholin's glands adjacent to the vaginal orifice. Frequently, the mucosa of the distal rectum is also involved in the inflammatory process. Some women with gonorrhea have few or no symptoms but nevertheless are highly infectious to male sexual contacts.

Sometimes the gonorrheal infection spreads from the cervix through the uterus into the fallopian tubes, causing an *acute salpingitis*. This is usually characterized by abdominal pain, tenderness, fever, and leukocytosis. Sometimes the inflammatory process results in development of an abscess within the fallopian tube or an abscess involving both the tube and the adjacent ovary.

Diseases of the Cervix

Nonspecific chronic cervicitis is a common mild inflammatory process involving the epithelium of the endocervix. It usually has little clinical significance.

Squamous cell carcinoma of the cervix is also common. The tumor often remains localized within the epithelium of the cervix (in situ carcinoma) for a relatively long period of time. Eventually the tumor becomes invasive and may extend into the adjacent rectum and bladder by direct extension. The ureters, which lie on each side of the cervix, may also be invaded and obstructed by a cervical carcinoma. Metastatic spread to distant sites is also relatively common. The Papanicolaou smear method is widely used by physicians to detect early cervical carcinoma. If the tumor is recognized and treated when it is still confined to the epithelium of the cervix, the cure rate approaches 100 per cent.

Diseases of the Endometrium and Myometrium

Occasionally the endometrium of the uterus may undergo *hyperplasia*, frequently associated with irregular uterine bleeding. *Endometrial adeno-carcinoma* is less frequent than cervical carcinoma and is also manifested by irregular uterine bleeding or postmenopausal bleeding. Benign smooth-muscle tumors, called *myomas*, which arise in the wall of the uterus, are frequently encountered; they are said to occur in approximately 30 per cent of women over 30 years of age. Occasionally myomas may be responsible for excessive or irregular uterine bleeding or may produce symptoms due to pressure on the adjacent bladder or rectum. Treatment consists of removal of the uterus (hysterectomy) if the myomas are producing symptoms.

Diseases of the Fallopian Tube

Acute salpingitis frequently develops as a complication of gonorrhea, as discussed. Acute tubal inflammation may also be caused by various other bacteria. Both gonorrheal and nongonorrheal salpingitis respond to appropriate antibiotic therapy. However, healing of the inflammatory process may be associated with scarring and obstruction of the lumen of the tube. Sterility may ensue if the obstruction is bilateral. Occasionally, even if the tubes are not completely occluded, the scarring may cause a delay in the transport of the fertilized ovum through the tube and lead to implantation of the ovum in the fallopian tube rather than in the endometrial cavity.

Diseases of the Ovary

CYSTS AND TUMORS

Benign cysts derived from ovarian follicles or corpora lutea occur frequently. Benign cystic teratomas, often called *dermoid cysts*, are also common in the ovary, as described in Chapter 12. These tumors may include teeth, bone, portions of brain, gastrointestinal tract, thyroid, and other tissues growing in a jumbled fashion. It has been said that the dermoid cyst reproduces imperfectly the structure of a fetus. However, ovarian tissue has the potential of giving rise to many types of tissue. Therefore, the dermoid cyst is more properly considered as a manifestation of the potential present in tumor cells as well as in normal ovarian tissue.

A number of different types of carcinoma also arise in the ovary, but these are much less frequent than malignant tumors of the cervix or endometrium.

ENDOMETRIOSIS

Endometriosis refers to the presence of endometrium in any location outside of the endometrial cavity. Occasionally ectopic deposits of endometrium may be encountered in the wall of the uterus, in the ovary, or elsewhere in the pelvis. Sometimes endometrial tissue is found in the appendix or in the rectum. These deposits respond to normal hormonal stimuli and therefore undergo cyclic menstrual desquamation and regeneration. Since the misplaced endometrial tissue does not communicate with the endometrial cavity, the "menstruating" tissue is not discharged through the vagina. Old blood and desquamated material are retained in the ectopic sites, leading to considerable scarring and a variety of clinical symptoms. Obstruction of the fallopian tubes by scar tissue may cause sterility.

Chapter 21

Diseases Associated
with Pregnancy

NORMAL PREGNANCY begins with the fertilization of the ovum in the fallopian tube. The fertilized ovum traverses the tube and implants itself in the endometrial cavity. After fertilization, the ovum undergoes progressive cell division and differentiates into two major groups of cells. One group of cells eventually gives rise to the fetus. The other cells give rise to the fetal membranes and placenta. When the fertilized ovum has burrowed into the endometrial cavity, a network of villi begins to develop, designed to derive nourishment from the maternal bloodstream and carry it to the growing embryo. In the process of growth and differentiation of the fetus and the placenta, a separate network of fetal blood vessels and blood cells evolves within the villi. Growth and differentiation of the fetus and placenta continue throughout pregnancy. Eventually the fetus lies within a fluid-filled sac within the uterus, connected to the placenta by the umbilical cord. The placenta is a large mass of villi lying in close contact with large maternal blood channels within the lining of the uterus. Blood from the fetus is circulated through the umbilical cord to the placenta, where it passes through the vascular channels in the placental villi. The fetal blood receives oxygen and nutrients from the maternal bloodstream by diffusion across the placental villi. The maternal circulation also excretes waste products from the fetus which diffuse from the fetal bloodstream into the maternal circulation. Normally, no intermixing of fetal and maternal bloodstreams occurs. They remain two separate and distinct circulations.

Spontaneous Abortion ("Miscarriage")

About 10 per cent of all pregnancies are estimated to terminate in spontaneous abortion. This generally occurs in early pregnancy, probably due

112

to defective implantation of the fertilized ovum or abnormalities in cell division of the ovum during the critical early stages of development. In most cases, the cause of the spontaneous abortion in early pregnancy cannot be determined. Occasionally, intrauterine fetal death occurs late in pregnancy. This is generally caused by partial detachment of the placenta from the wall of the uterus, or by obstruction of the blood supply through the umbilical cord. Compression of the blood vessels in the umbilical cord (shutting off the blood supply to the fetus) may occur if the cord becomes knotted or wrapped tightly around the infant's neck, arm, or leg. If the placenta becomes separated or the cord becomes obstructed, the fetus no longer receives oxygen and nutrients from the mother and it dies. Usually a dead fetus is expelled promptly, but occasionally it is retained within the uterine cavity for several weeks or months.

If a dead fetus is retained for some time within the uterine cavity, products of degenerated fetal tissue diffuse into the maternal circulation. This material has thromboplastic activity and may induce a hemorrhagic disease in the mother due to depletion of maternal blood coagulation factors. This is the result of activation of the coagulation mechanism by the thromboplastic material. A retained dead fetus is one cause of *disseminated intravascular coagulation,* which has been discussed in the section on blood coagulation (Chapter 13).

Ectopic Pregnancy

An ectopic pregnancy (*ecto* = outside) is the development of an embryo outside of its normal location within the uterine cavity. Most ectopic pregnancies occur in the fallopian tubes, but rarely a fertilized ovum may develop in the ovary or abdominal cavity. Normally, fertilization occurs in the fallopian tube, and the fertilized ovum then proceeds into the endometrial cavity where implantation occurs. Occasionally, the fertilized ovum may be impeded in its progress through the tube, and implantation will occur within the fallopian tubes. The fallopian tube is not equipped to sustain the rapidly growing fetus and membranes. The tube becomes distended and eventually ruptures, often causing severe bleeding.

Hydatidiform Mole

Occasionally the chorionic villi do not develop normally, but become converted into large, cystic structures resembling masses of grapes. The cells making up the villi may also proliferate excessively. The proliferating cells may infiltrate the wall of the uterus, causing hemorrhage and occasionally leading to perforation of the uterus.

Choriocarcinoma

Choriocarcinoma is a rare malignant tumor which develops from the proliferating cells of the placental villi. The tumor invades the wall of the uterus and may metastasize to distant sites. In this case, the malignant tumor is derived not from the maternal cells, but from the cells of the placenta.

Hemolytic Disease of the Newborn (Erythroblastosis Fetalis)

Erythroblastosis fetalis is a hemolytic anemia in the newborn infant resulting from sensitization of the mother to a "foreign" blood-group antigen present in the red cells of the fetus. The mother reacts by forming antibody which crosses the placenta and damages the infant's red cells, resulting in accelerated destruction of the red cells. The infant attempts to "keep up" with the increased blood destruction by increasing the rate of red cell production (compensatory hematopoiesis). The severity of the hemolytic disease depends on the intensity of the blood destruction in the infant. If the hemolytic process is extremely marked, the infant often dies in the uterus during the last trimester of pregnancy. The severely affected infant has marked anemia and is very edematous. This severe form of erythroblastosis is often called *hydrops fetalis*, the term "hydrops" referring to the severe edema in the affected infant. The edema is due to heart failure as well as impaired plasma protein synthesis by the liver, both of which result from the severe anemia. If the hemolytic process is less intense, the infant may be born alive but will be moderately or severely anemic. Infants with mild disease may appear normal at birth but become anemic and jaundiced soon afterward.

CHANGES IN HEMOGLOBIN AND BILIRUBIN AFTER DELIVERY

Figure 21-1 illustrates the typical changes in hemoglobin and bilirubin levels in an infant with hemolytic disease after delivery. Anemia invariably develops or increases in severity after delivery; jaundice also develops rapidly. Aggravation of the anemia is due to a decline in the rate of compensatory hematopoiesis following delivery. In the uterus, hematopoiesis is stimulated by both the increased blood destruction and the low oxygen tension in the fetal blood. After delivery, respiration is established, and the arterial oxygen tension in the infant's blood rises. The stimulus to hematopoiesis induced by the low intrauterine oxygen tension is no longer present, and the rate of compensatory hematopoiesis declines. However, blood destruction continues at the same rate. The increase in

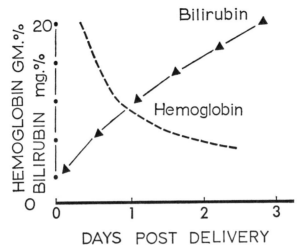

Fig. 21-1.—Changes in hemoglobin and bilirubin concentration in infant with hemolytic disease after delivery.

the degree of anemia reflects the greater postnatal disproportion between blood production and blood destruction.

Jaundice in hemolytic disease is also due to the accelerated blood destruction. The increased rate of red cell breakdown leads to production of large amounts of bile pigment. Before delivery, the bile pigment crosses the placenta into the maternal circulation and is excreted by the mother. After delivery, the infant is called upon to excrete the large amount of pigment previously handled by the mother. However, the liver of the newborn infant is still relatively inefficient in conjugating and excreting bilirubin. As a result, the level of unconjugated bilirubin rises rapidly in the infant's blood. This is hazardous to the infant because high levels of unconjugated bilirubin are toxic to the nervous system, causing necrosis and degeneration of brain tissue (called *kernicterus*).

Most cases of hemolytic disease are due to maternal-fetal Rh incompatibility. The Rh system is a relatively complex blood group system composed of many antigens. However, the most important Rh antigen clinically is the Rh_o *antigen*. (The subscript "o" refers to "original," meaning that this was the first Rh antigen recognized.) The Rh_o antigen is also called the *D antigen*. For clinical purposes, a patient is considered Rh-positive if this antigen is present and Rh-negative if it is absent, no matter what other Rh antigens are present. In the vast majority of cases of hemolytic disease, the patient is Rh_o (D) negative, the infant is Rh_o (D) positive, and the antibody is anti-Rh_o (anti-D). However, hemolytic disease may occasionally result from sensitization of the mother to another antigen in the Rh system, or from sensitization to an antigen in one of the other blood group systems. The essential feature required for the pathogenesis of hemolytic disease is maternal-fetal blood-group incompatibility, and this may be due to any of a number of blood-group antigens.

DIAGNOSIS OF HEMOLYTIC DISEASE IN THE NEWBORN INFANT

From a knowledge of the pathogenesis of the disease, it follows that the diagnosis of hemolytic disease can be made when the following features are demonstrated (Table 21-1):

(1) Blood-group differences between mother and child. The child has a blood-group antigen lacking in the mother's blood. In the most common type of hemolytic disease, the mother lacks the Rh_o (D) antigen, which is present in the cells of the infant.

(2) Sensitization of the mother to the "foreign" antigen in the infant's cells. This involves demonstrating the presence of an antibody in the mother's blood directed against the "foreign" antigen. Usually this is anti-Rh_o (D).

(3) Passage of antibody across the placenta into the infant's blood, with fixation of the antibody to the surface of the infant's cells. This is demonstrated by means of the direct Coombs' test performed on the infant's blood. This test detects antibody protein coating on the surface of the infant's red cells.

(4) Evidence of increased destruction of the infant's cells. Determination of the hemoglobin and bilirubin levels in the infant's blood indicates the intensity of the hemolytic process.

When these criteria have been met, the diagnosis of hemolytic disease is established with certainty. In routine clinical practice, this information can be obtained rapidly without great difficulty. Generally, blood-typing of the mother and studies to determine the presence of antibodies are

TABLE 21-1.—DIAGNOSIS OF HEMOLYTIC DISEASE

CHARACTERISTIC FEATURE	MEANS OF RECOGNITION
Production on antigenic fetal cells	Maternal-fetal blood-group differences; mother lacks antigen present in fetal cells
Maternal sensitization	Mother's blood contains antibody against antigenic cells
Transplacental passage of maternal antibody	Positive direct Coombs' test on cord blood
Increased blood destruction in newborn infant	Decreased hemoglobin in cord blood; elevated bilirubin

performed routinely by the physician during pregnancy, and he generally knows before delivery whether the mother has been sensitized and is likely to deliver an affected infant. When the infant is born, a sample of blood from the umbilical cord (which is the infant's blood) is sent to the laboratory for determination of blood type and direct Coombs' test, as well as hemoglobin and bilirubin levels. The Coombs' test and blood type indicate whether the infant is affected, and the hemoglobin and bilirubin levels indicate the severity of the hemolytic disease.

TREATMENT OF HEMOLYTIC DISEASE

The most common and widely used treatment of erythroblastosis is *exchange transfusion*. The infant with hemolytic disease is in jeopardy because his body is saturated with passively transferred maternal antibody. The antibody is the cause of the hemolytic anemia and jaundice, and several months are required before the antibody can be completely eliminated from the infant's circulation. The rationale of exchange transfusion is to provide the infant with a population of cells which will not be destroyed by the antibody. In the usual case of hemolytic disease due to Rh_o incompatibility, a transfusion of Rh-negative blood is given. At the same time, exchange transfusion provides the infant with bilirubin-free plasma to replace the jaundiced plasma, thereby helping to prevent marked elevation of potentially toxic, unconjugated bilirubin. It should be emphasized that the exchange transfusion has no effect on the infant's own blood type. The transfused Rh-negative cells will be gradually eliminated and replaced by the infant's own Rh-positive cells. The purpose of the exchange transfusion is to tide the infant over an acute life-threatening situation. This is accomplished by decreasing the rate of red cell destruction through transfusion of cells not subject to hemolysis, and by lowering the concentration of potentially toxic unconjugated bilirubin in the infant's plasma.

Exchange transfusion may be compared to replacing the contents of a barrel of salt water with fresh water without emptying and refilling the barrel. This can be accomplished by withdrawing a pail of salt water from the barrel and replacing an equal quantity of fresh water. If this is repeated many times, the salt concentration of the water in the barrel is gradually reduced until eventually the barrel is filled with fresh water. An exchange transfusion involves the same principle. The usual method of exchange transfusion is to introduce a catheter into the umbilical vein. A small quantity of the infant's own blood is withdrawn and replaced with an equal quantity of blood lacking the sensitizing antigen (usually Rh-negative blood). The process of withdrawing a small quantity of blood and replacing it with an equal quantity of exchange blood is continued until about 500 ml of blood has been administered. At the conclusion of the exchange transfusion, about 85 per cent of the infant's own cells will have been replaced by the transfused cells.

INTRAUTERINE FETAL TRANSFUSION

Exchange transfusion can be used to treat only those infants who survive long enough to be born alive. It cannot be used to salvage severely affected infants who often die in utero late in pregnancy. Recently, a method has been found which can identify fetuses severely affected with erythroblastosis. A needle is inserted through the maternal abdominal wall, through the uterus, and into the amnionic cavity, and a small quantity of amnionic fluid is withdrawn. The amnionic fluid of infants affected with hemolytic disease often contains increased amounts of bile pigments; a rough correlation exists between the severity of the hemolytic disease and the amount of pigments in the amnionic fluid. If the study of the fluid indicates that the infant is severely affected and may not survive, it is possible to administer a blood transfusion to the fetus while it is still within the uterus. It is not necessary to inject the blood into a vein. Blood can be introduced into the infant's peritoneal cavity and will be adequately absorbed. This method requires highly specialized technics and carries a risk to the infant. It is used only in extremely desperate situations where the infant is likely to die if transfusion is not performed.

RH-IMMUNE GLOBULIN

A recent development shows great promise in preventing hemolytic disease due to Rh incompatibility. Shortly after delivery, gamma globulin containing potent Rh antibody is administered to unsensitized Rh-negative mothers who have given birth to Rh-positive infants. Apparently the passively transferred gamma globulin suppresses or prevents antibody formation by the mother, thereby preventing sensitization. It is also likely that the passively transferred antibody destroys any Rh-positive cells from the infant which may have gotten into the mother's circulation at the time of delivery. The rapid removal of these cells decreases the likelihood of sensitization.

FACTORS INFLUENCING THE FREQUENCY OF HEMOLYTIC DISEASE

One question frequently asked is why Rh hemolytic disease is not more common. Rh incompatibility between husband and wife is present in about 10 per cent of all marriages. However, Rh hemolytic disease is encountered in less than 1 per cent of all pregnancies. This is because sensitization of the Rh-negative mother generally requires more than one Rh-positive pregnancy. Many Rh-incompatible matings involve Rh-positive heterozygous husbands, so that some of the infants will be Rh-negative and will cause no sensitization. In addition, some individuals are not good "antibody-formers" and require several contacts with Rh-positive blood before developing antibodies. Another factor influencing sensitization is the ABO groups of the mother and infant. If the ABO group of the infant is incompatible with the ABO antibodies in the maternal blood (for example, infant group A and mother group O with anti-A and anti-B antibodies), any fetal cells introduced into the maternal circulation at the time of delivery will be destroyed by the maternal ABO antibodies. Therefore, the Rh-positive fetal cells are unable to circulate long enough to induce sensitization. On the other hand, if the ABO group of the infant is compatible with the ABO antibodies in the maternal serum (for example, both mother and infant of the same ABO group, or group O infant whose cells would be compatible with any maternal ABO group), the Rh-positive infant's cells would persist in the maternal circulation for several months and would be much more likely to provoke sensitization.

ABO Hemolytic Disease

In most cases, hemolytic diseases of infants is the result of sensitization to a "foreign" antigen, which provokes the formation of a new antibody. However, a very mild type of hemolytic disease occasionally may be due to ABO blood group differences between mother and infant. In this situation, the mother is group O (and has anti-A and anti-B antibodies in her serum) and the infant is either group A or group B. The A or B antigen of the fetus stimulates the maternal ABO antibodies, increasing the titer and changing the character of the antibodies, so that they are capable of crossing the placenta and becoming fixed to the cells of the infant. ABO hemolytic disease may be encountered in a first pregnancy, since it is due to a preexisting antibody capable of being stimulated by an ABO-incompatible pregnancy. This is in contrast to most other types of hemolytic disease, in which a first pregnancy is required to provoke sensitization before antibody can be formed in a subsequent pregnancy.

Chapter 22

The Urinary System

THE KIDNEY is an important excretory organ, functioning along with the lung in excreting the products of the metabolism of food. Carbon dioxide and water are end products of carbohydrate and fat metabolism. Protein metabolism is associated with the production of urea and various acids, in addition. These two waste products can be excreted only by the kidneys. The kidney also plays an important role in the regulation of mineral and water balance. This is accomplished by excretion of minerals and water that have been ingested in excess of the body's requirements, or by conservation of minerals and water when necessary. It has been said that the internal environment of the body is determined not by what the person ingests but rather by what the kidneys retain. The kidney serves an endocrine function, as well. Certain specialized cells in the kidney elaborate humoral substances which regulate red blood cell production in the bone marrow (erythropoietin) and other substances concerned with the regulation of the blood pressure (renin).

The basic structural unit of the kidney is the *nephron*. It consists of a *glomerulus* and a *renal tubule*. The glomerulus consists of a capillary tuft supplied by an *afferent glomerular artery*. The capillaries of the glomerulus then recombine into an *efferent glomerular artery*, which supplies blood to the renal tubule. The glomerulus is invaginated into the end of the tubule and is covered by a thin layer of epithelial cells derived from the tubule. The glomeruli are concerned with the nonselective filtration of water and soluble materials from the blood passing through the glomerular tufts. The tubules selectively reabsorb water, minerals, and other substances which are conserved by the body. They also actively secrete unwanted materials directly into the tubular lumens. The urine excreted by the kidneys represents the glomerular filtrate after most of the water and important constituents have been reabsorbed by the renal tubules, to which has been added other metabolites excreted by the renal tubules (Fig. 22-1). From a consideration of normal glomerular and tubular func-

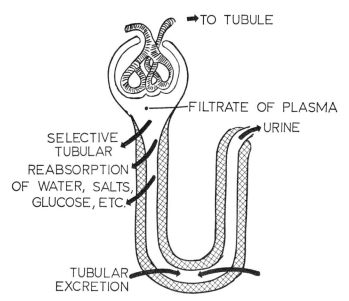

Fig. 22-1.—Basic concepts of glomerular and tubular function.

tion, it follows that normal renal function requires a free flow of blood through the afferent glomerular arterioles, normal glomerular capillaries, normal permeability of the glomerular basement membranes, normal tubular function, and normal urinary drainage structures to convey urine from the kidney to the bladder and out the urethra. Derangement of any of these functions results in renal disease.

Glomerulonephritis

As the term implies, *glomerulonephritis* is an inflammation of the renal glomeruli. Glomerulonephritis represents not a bacterial infection, but a hypersensitivity state induced after infection with some strains of beta hemolytic streptococci. The pathogenesis of glomerulonephritis resembles that of rheumatic fever in many ways; particularly, a delayed hypersensitivity to beta streptococci is involved. In glomerulonephritis, the hypersensitivity is manifested by swelling and inflammation of the renal glomeruli and injury to the glomerular basement membrane. Many of the glomeruli become completely obstructed by swelling and cellular infiltration; other glomeruli are damaged and their ability to act as a selective filter is impaired, leading to leakage of red cells and protein into the urine.

The signs and symptoms of glomerulonephritis are related to the changes within the glomeruli. Since many glomeruli are completely blocked by inflammation, less blood is filtered and less urine is excreted. With the reduction of urinary output, waste products are retained and accumulate in the blood. The urine contains large numbers of red cells and protein. Frequently masses of cells and protein become trapped within the tubules and molded into the shape of the renal tubules before being excreted in the urine. These are called *urinary casts* and are an important indication of renal injury.

In most cases, the inflammatory process subsides and the patient recovers completely without residual kidney damage. Occasionally, the disease is so severe that the patient dies of renal insufficiency. In some patients, the glomerulonephritis never heals completely. The disease becomes chronic and progresses slowly, eventually leading to renal failure. Patients with chronic glomerulonephritis may suffer recurrent episodes of acute nephritis after beta streptococcal infection. This is analogous to the situation in rheumatic fever, in which recurrent beta streptococcal infections are followed by recurrent episodes of rheumatic fever.

Arteriolar Nephrosclerosis

This disease (sometimes called simply *nephrosclerosis*) is a complication of severe hypertension. Because of the marked elevation of the systemic blood pressure, the small arterioles and arteries throughout the body are called upon to carry blood at a much higher pressure than normal. As a result, the blood vessels undergo severe degenerative changes characterized by thickening and narrowing of the lumens; this reduces blood flow through the narrowed arterioles. The name of the disease, which means literally "sclerosis of the arterioles of the nephrons," refers to these characteristic renal vascular changes. Glomerular filtration is reduced because of the marked arteriolar narrowing. The renal tubules, which are also supplied by the glomerular arterioles, also undergo degenerative changes. Patients with severe nephrosclerosis may die from renal insufficiency, as well as from the effects of the severe hypertension.

Cystitis

Cystitis is a bacterial infection of the bladder, either acute or chronic. The patient complains of burning pain on urination and usually has a desire to urinate frequently. These symptoms are due to the congestion and inflammation of the bladder mucosa. Cystitis is generally not serious, but the infection may spread into the upper urinary passages, involving the renal pelvis and kidney. Cystitis is somewhat more common in women than men, probably because the short urethra allows easier access of organisms into the bladder.

Pyelonephritis

In contrast to glomerulonephritis, pyelonephritis is an actual bacterial infection of the kidney. The term refers to the involvement of both the renal pelvis and the renal tissue in the inflammatory process (*pyelo* = pelvis + *nephritis* = kidney inflammation). Bacteria usually infect the kidney by ascending upward from the lower urinary tract (*ascending pyelonephritis*), but occasionally the organisms may be carried to the kidney through the bloodstream (*hematogenous pyelonephritis*). Any factors impairing urinary drainage will predispose a patient to pyelonephritis, because stagnation of urine tends to promote multiplication of bacteria gaining access to the urine by ascending up the urethra. Stones developing anywhere in the urinary system may also predispose one to infection.

The symptoms of pyelonephritis are those of any acute infection, together with localized pain and tenderness over the affected kidney. Since cystitis and pyelonephritis are frequently associated, the patient usually experiences urinary frequency and pain on urination, as well. Large numbers of white blood cells and bacteria are found in the urine. The patient is treated with appropriate antibiotics, together with measures directed at correcting any abnormalities in the lower urinary tract which may impede drainage of urine and predispose to infection.

Most episodes of pyelonephritis are acute and self-limited. The body is capable of overcoming the infection, and the damaged areas in the kidney heal by scarring. The main danger of pyelonephritis lies in the tendency of the disease to become chronic and recurrent. With each subsequent attack, more kidney tissue is destroyed, resulting in healing by scarring. After many episodes of infection, the kidney may become markedly scarred and shrunken, and the patient may eventually develop symptoms of renal insufficiency.

Nephrotic Syndrome

The term *nephrotic syndrome* refers to a group of abnormalities characterized by marked loss of protein in the urine, leading to a reduction of proteins in the blood plasma. This, in turn, causes marked edema due to the low plasma osmotic pressure (Chapter 14). The syndrome may be produced by a number of different types of renal diseases. The basic cause is injury to the glomerulus, allowing leakage of protein through the damaged basement membrane. Since the albumin molecule is much smaller than the globulin molecule, a disproportionately large amount of albumin is lost in the urine. The osmotic pressure of the plasma is markedly decreased, allowing excessive transudation of fluid from the capillaries into the interstitial tissues and body cavities. Patients with the nephrotic syndrome have marked leg edema, and often fluid collects in the abdominal cavity (called *ascites*); sometimes fluid also accumulates in the pleural cavities (called *hydrothorax*).

The nephrotic syndrome is most common in children and is due to relatively minimal glomerular basement membrane injury of undetermined cause. In most children, the disease lasts from 1 to 3 years; the majority of children recover completely. In contrast to the favorable outcome in children, the nephrotic syndrome in the adult is usually a manifestation of progressive, more serious renal disease. Some cases are examples of chronic progressive glomerulonephritis; others are a manifestation of a collagen disease (such as lupus erythematosus) affecting the kidney. Some other relatively uncommon types of kidney disease involving the glomeruli may also produce this syndrome.

Renal Tubular Injury

The blood supply to the renal tubules is derived from the efferent glomerular artery, and minor degrees of tubular injury are seen in many diseases involving the renal glomeruli. Renal tubular injury in the absence of glomerular disease may be encountered in two situations: (1) tubular necrosis due to impaired renal blood flow, and (2) tubular necrosis due to toxic drugs and chemicals. In the former situation, any condition associated with shock and marked drop in the blood pressure leads to impaired blood flow to the kidneys. This is often manifested by degeneration and necrosis of renal tubules. In the latter case, various drugs and chemicals are excreted by the kidneys and cause direct toxic injury to the tubular epithelium.

The major clinical feature of tubular necrosis is a marked decrease in urine output (*oliguria*) or complete suppression of urine formation (*anuria*). This occurs when the damaged tubular epithelium has lost its capacity for selective tubular reabsorption, and the glomerular filtrate diffuses back through the damaged tubular epithelium into the adjacent peritubular blood vessels. After a period of several weeks, tubular function is slowly restored by regeneration of the damaged epithelium, but several months may be required before renal function returns completely to normal. During the period of anuria, renal dialysis by means of an artificial kidney can be used to maintain the patient until tubular function has been restored.

Urinary Tract Obstruction

After urine has been formed by the kidneys, it must be excreted through the ureters into the bladder and out the urethra. If the outflow of urine is obstructed at any point, the ureters gradually dilate (*hydroureter*) as does the renal pelvis (*hydronephrosis*) proximal to the area of obstruction. Eventually, the kidneys become atrophic as a result of accumulation of urine under increased pressure proximal to the obstruction. The hydronephrosis may involve one or both kidneys. If outflow of urine from the bladder is obstructed, hydronephrosis will be bilateral. The hydronephrosis will be unilateral if obstruction involves only one ureter. Enlargement of the prostate, common in elderly men, is a frequent cause of urinary tract obstruction. However, obstruction may be due to a large number of causes, such as a tumor in the bladder or ureter or a kidney stone that has become impacted in the ureter.

Conditions leading to hydronephrosis also cause retention and stagnation of urine. This, in turn, may produce further complications. Stagnation of urine predisposes a patient to infection, causing cystitis and pyelonephritis. Stagnation also predisposes one to stone formation due to precipitation of urinary salts. A cycle may become established in which hydronephrosis predisposes to stone and infection; these, in turn, may increase the degree of urinary tract obstruction and cause further progression of the hydronephrosis.

Renal Cysts

Solitary cysts of the kidney are relatively common, varying in size from a few millimeters up to about 15 cm in diameter. They are not associated with impairment in renal function and are of no significance to the patient.

Congenital polycystic kidney is a hereditary abnormality transmitted as a mendelian dominant trait, characterized by the formation of multiple cysts throughout the kidney. Apparently it is due to abnormal development of the renal tubule and collecting tubule systems. The cysts enlarge progressively, gradually replacing normal renal tissue and eventually leading to renal insufficiency. The age at which the cysts cause renal failure depends upon the rapidity with which the cysts enlarge. In some cases, polycystic kidneys cause renal functional impairment in newborn infants and young children. In other cases, the disease progresses more slowly, and renal insufficiency does not appear until young adulthood or even late middle age.

Tumors of the Urinary Tract

Both benign and malignant tumors may arise from the kidney or from the epithelium of the bladder, ureters, or renal pelvis. Rarely, an unusual malignant tumor occurs in the kidney of infants and young children. This apparently arises from persisting embryonic tissue, and the tumor somewhat resembles the structure of the embryonic kidney; it is called a *nephroblastoma* or *Wilms' tumor* (Chapter 12).

Evaluation of Renal Disease by the Physician

The physician uses several methods to detect renal disease, to evaluate the extent of disturbance of renal function, and to define the type of renal disease.

Examination of the urine is a valuable method for detecting the presence or absence of renal disease. The presence of red cells and protein in the urine indicates damage to the glomerulus, allowing leakage of these substances into the glomerular filtrate. Renal casts, which are collections of protein and cells molded in the shape of the kidney tubules, are also indicative of glomerular disease.

Impaired renal function can be recognized by measuring the levels of various substances, such as urea, which are normally excreted by the kidney. Elevated levels indicate impairment of renal function, and the degree of elevation above normal is a rough measure of the severity of the renal disease.

The degree of impairment of renal function can then be evaluated by means of a number of renal function tests. These tests measure the ability of the kidneys to remove various substances from the blood and excrete them in the urine. They provide rough quantitative information concerning the degree of impairment of renal function. Renal function tests are often used to follow the course of a patient with renal disease.

Many times the physician cannot make an exact diagnosis concerning the type of renal disease without resorting to biopsy of the kidney and histologic examination of kidney tissue. This can be accomplished without undue difficulty or risk to the patient by introducing a small biopsy needle through the skin of the flank directly into the substance of the kidney. A small bit of kidney tissue is removed for histologic study. Examination of the biopsy material by the pathologist often permits an exact diagnosis as to the nature and extent of the renal disease; this serves as a guide to proper treatment.

Renal Failure (Uremia)

Renal failure represents the end stage of any type of chronic renal disease. It becomes apparent when the kidneys are no longer able to perform their normal regulatory and excretory functions. The patient experiences severe derangements of electrolyte and acid-base balance due to loss of the kidneys' regulatory functions. In addition, various acids and minerals are retained which would normally be excreted by the kidneys. The term *uremia* refers to the characteristic retention of urea in the blood in renal failure. Urea is a product of protein metabolism normally excreted by the kidneys. It is not toxic, but the level of urea in the blood correlates roughly with the degree of retention of other waste products. Therefore, the concentration of urea in the blood is often used as a rough measure of the severity of renal failure.

The symptoms of uremia are nonspecific. They consist of weakness and usually moderate anemia. Eventually the patient has convulsions, lapses into coma, and dies. Until recently, there was no effective treatment; however, the development of artificial kidney machines has permitted individuals with uremia to be maintained in reasonably good health for long periods of time. In certain selected patients, the diseased kidneys can be replaced by transplantation of kidneys from a normal healthy donor (Chapter 3).

Chapter 23

The Male Reproductive System

THE COMPONENTS of the male reproductive system are the penis, the prostate and certain accessory glands, the testes, and a duct system for transporting sperm from the testes to the urethra. The transport duct system consists of the epididymis, which is closely applied to the testes, and continues as the vas deferens (plural term is "vasa deferentia"). The two vasa extend upward in the spermatic cords and enter the prostatic urethra as the ejaculatory ducts. The urethra is divided into a long penile urethra and a short segment transversing the prostate gland, called the prostatic urethra. It is conventional to speak of the distal penile urethra as the "anterior urethra," and the prostatic urethra and adjacent proximal part of the penile urethra as the "posterior urethra." Figure 23-1 illustrates the anatomy of the male reproductive system. A working knowledge of how these structures are interrelated is necessary in order to understand the spread of inflammatory disease in the male reproductive tract and the various complications that may result.

Fig. 23-1.—The interrelationship of the various components of the male reproductive system, viewed from the posterior surface.

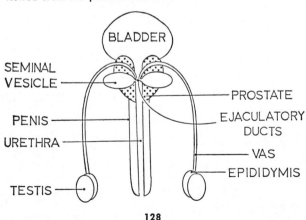

Gonorrhea

Gonorrhea is a relatively common disease. The gonococcus, spread by sexual contact, initially causes an acute inflammation of the anterior urethra. However, the inflammation may spread into the posterior urethra, prostate, seminal vesicles, and epididymides. The gonococcus may also cause an acute inflammation of the rectal mucosa. Occasionally, healing of the gonorrheal inflammation in the posterior urethra may be associated with considerable scarring, leading to narrowing of the urethra and urinary tract obstruction. Inflammatory obstruction of the vasa deferentia may block sperm transport and lead to sterility.

Chronic Prostatitis

Mild, nonspecific inflammation of the prostate gland is common and produces relatively few clinical symptoms.

Benign Prostatic Hyperplasia

Moderate enlargement of the prostate gland is relatively common in elderly men. Prostatic enlargement is significant only if it obstructs the bladder neck, leading to incomplete emptying of the bladder, or causes complete urinary tract obstruction. An enlarged obstructing prostate causes difficulty in urinating and may lead to various other complications due to urinary retention and stagnation of urine in the bladder, such as cystitis, pyelonephritis, hydronephrosis, and stone formation. Treatment consists of surgical resection of the enlarged portions of gland blocking the neck of the bladder.

Tumors

Carcinoma of the Prostate

Carcinoma of the prostate is a relatively common tumor in elderly men. The initial symptoms are usually due to urinary tract obstruction resulting from the encroachment of the tumor-infiltrated prostate on the neck of the bladder. Most prostatic carcinomas are dependent on male sex hormones for their continued growth. Therefore, many prostatic tumors can be treated effectively either by removal of the testes surgically, which eradicates the source of male sex hormone, or by the administration of female sex hormone. Either castration or hormone treatment usually causes regression of the tumor.

CARCINOMA OF THE TESTIS

Carcinoma of the testis is uncommon and occurs in young men. Some testicular tumors elaborate chorionic gonadotrophic hormones (the same type of hormones produced by the placenta in pregnancy). Therefore, some patients with testicular tumors have a positive "pregnancy test" due to the chorionic gonadotrophins secreted by the tumor.

CARCINOMA OF THE PENIS

Carcinoma of the penis is also uncommon; it is almost never encountered in a circumcised male. It is generally considered that the secretions which accumulate under the foreskin of the penis are carcinogenic and that this accumulation is prevented by circumcision. However, other factors may also account for the low incidence of carcinoma in circumcised males.

Chapter 24

The Liver and Biliary System

THE LIVER, located in the upper abdomen, is the largest organ in the body. It weighs about 1,500 gm. It is a complex organ with many functions. These are concerned primarily with metabolism of ingested carbohydrates, protein, and fat delivered via the portal circulation, synthesis of various substances including plasma proteins and proteins concerned with blood clotting, storage of vitamin B_{12} and other materials, and detoxification and excretion of various substances.

The basic structural unit is the liver lobule. Each lobule consists of cords of cells radiating outward from a central vein. The liver has a double blood supply, being supplied both by the hepatic artery and portal vein. The hepatic artery supplies oxygenated arterial blood. The portal vein supplies venous blood collected from the gastrointestinal tract. Both the hepatic artery and portal vein divide into numerous branches within the liver; they empty into sinusoids which lie between the liver cords. The sinusoidal blood eventually empties into the central vein of the lobule. The central veins gradually join to form the hepatic veins and ultimately empty into the inferior vena cava.

From the liver, two hepatic ducts unite to form the common hepatic duct. This is joined by the gallbladder and cystic duct to form the common bile duct, which empties into the duodenum. Bile is stored and concentrated in the gallbladder.

Bile

FORMATION AND EXCRETION

Bile pigment is a product of the breakdown of red cells. Red cells normally survive about 4 months. The worn-out erythrocytes are broken down by the reticuloendothelial cells throughout the body. The iron derived from the hemoglobin is conserved by the body and reused for synthesis of new hemoglobin. The iron-free pigment is bilirubin. Since

131

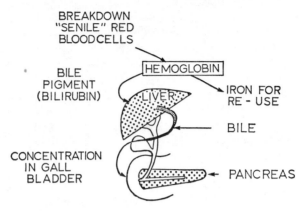

Fig. 24-1.—Formation and excretion of bile.

the breakdown of red cells proceeds in reticuloendothelial tissues through-out the body, small quantities of bile pigment are present continually in the blood. When the blood passes through the liver, the bilirubin is re-moved by the liver cells. Excretion is accomplished by combining the bilirubin with other substances, a process called *conjugation,* which re-quires certain specific enzymes. Most of the bilirubin is conjugated with glucuronic acid and excreted as bilirubin glucuronide. The conjugated bilirubin is much more soluble and less toxic than the unconjugated mate-rial. The bile pigment is excreted into the small bile channels between the liver cell cords; it is collected into large ducts at the periphery of the lobules which eventually unite to form the major bile ducts. Figure 24-1 summarizes the important concepts relating to the formation and excretion of bile.

COMPOSITION AND PROPERTIES

Bile consists of a mixture of substances excreted by the liver. In addi-tion to conjugated bilirubin, bile contains cholesterol, bile salts, water, minerals, and various other materials which have been detoxified by the liver cells and excreted. Bile is secreted continually and is concentrated and stored in the gallbladder. During digestion, the gallbladder contracts, squirting bile into the duodenum. Bile does not contain digestive en-zymes, but functions as a biologic detergent. Bile salts emulsify fat into small globules, increasing the surface area so that the fat can be acted upon more readily by pancreatic and duodenal enzymes. Digestion of fat is much less efficient in the absence of bile.

Liver Injury

The liver is vulnerable to injury by a large number of agents. Histologically, liver injury may be manifested by necrosis of liver cells, by accumulation of fat within the liver cell cytoplasm, or by a combination of the two. Some injurious agents cause primarily cell necrosis, whereas others induce chiefly fatty change in liver cells.

The effect of hepatic injury depends on the extent of damage induced by the injurious agent. If liver injury is mild, the liver cells will completely recover, restoring liver function to normal. Fortunately, this is the usual outcome. If the injury is extremely severe, large amounts of liver tissue are completely destroyed, and not enough liver may remain to sustain life. If the patient does survive, healing of the severe injury may be associated with marked scarring (postnecrotic scarring), and liver function may never return to normal. Multiple episodes of relatively mild liver injury may have a cumulative effect, leading to scarring and permanent impairment of liver function. Similarly, any chronic or progressive injury may cause scarring and impairment of function.

Fig. 24-2.—Summary of causes and effects of liver injury.

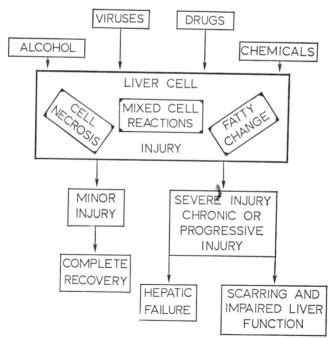

Liver cell injury caused by drugs, chemicals, alcohol, or toxins can also produce fatty change in liver cells rather than necrosis, as has been described. Prolonged fatty change may also impair hepatic function and lead eventually to scarring. Figure 24-2 diagrams the general causes and possible effects of various degrees of liver injury.

Clinically, the most common types of liver disease characterized by injury to liver cells are viral hepatitis, fatty liver, and cirrhosis of the liver.

Viral Hepatitis

Viral hepatitis is an acute inflammation of the liver due to a virus. Clinically, the disease is frequently associated with nausea, vomiting, discomfort and tenderness over the liver, and laboratory evidence of disturbed liver function. Jaundice is often present, reflecting the impaired ability of the liver cells to excrete bilirubin, but it may be absent in mild cases.

Two distinct types of viral hepatitis are recognized, due to two different viruses. One type is called *infectious hepatitis*, and the second is called *serum hepatitis*. These names were chosen to describe the usual methods of transmission of the two diseases. Although the viruses are different, the diseases are quite similar clinically, and it is impossible to determine which virus caused the hepatitis. The general term viral hepatitis refers to either type of virus-induced disease. In both types of viral hepatitis, the virus is present in the bloodstream of the infected individual during some stage of the disease.

INFECTIOUS HEPATITIS

In this type of viral hepatitis, the virus is excreted in the gastrointestinal tract, so that transmission usually occurs by the enteric route. Food or water is ingested which has been contaminated by virus excreted in the feces of an infected patient. However, since the virus is present in the bloodstream during the acute phase of the disease, infectious hepatitis can also be transmitted by blood transfusions, or by means of syringes, needles, or blood products contaminated by the virus. The incubation period is relatively short, and the disease is usually mild.

SERUM HEPATITIS

Serum hepatitis is usually transmitted by the parenteral route, that is, by a route other than the gastrointestinal tract. This is usually accomplished by means of transfusion of blood from a donor who is a carrier of the virus, although transmission is also possible by means of contaminated needles and syringes. The incubation period is much longer, and the disease tends to be more severe than infectious hepatitis.

These features distinguishing infectious hepatitis from serum hepatitis apply in most instances. However, exceptions do occur. As previously described, infectious hepatitis can be transmitted by blood transfusions or other parenteral means. There is also evidence that serum hepatitis may be transmitted by the enteric route, since hepatitis has developed in medical personnel caring for patients with serum hepatitis. Recently, outbreaks of both types of hepatitis among drug addicts have been traced to common use of contaminated needles or syringes.

COURSE OF VIRAL HEPATITIS

Viral hepatitis is one type of liver injury, and the comments made regarding the course and outcome of any liver injury also apply to viral hepatitis (Fig. 24-2). Fortunately, viral hepatitis is usually mild, and the majority of patients recover without complications. Some patients with mild disease do not become jaundiced, even though there is definite clinical and laboratory evidence of liver injury. This is called *anicteric hepatitis* (*ana* = without + *icterus* = jaundice). Some individuals infected with the virus have few symptoms, and the disease could easily escape detection (sometimes called "subclinical" hepatitis). An unfavorable outcome occurs only in a very small percentage of patients. Rarely, death may result from massive hepatic necrosis, or recovery from severe liver injury may be followed by persisting disability due to postnecrotic liver scarring. In a few patients, the disease becomes chronic and progressive, eventually leading to liver failure.

Some patients infected with hepatitis virus continue to harbor the virus in their blood for long periods of time, and some become chronic carriers of the virus. Such persons are capable of infecting other persons if their blood is introduced into another person by blood transfusion or by means of contaminated syringes.

AUSTRALIA ANTIGEN AND SERUM HEPATITIS

Recently, many patients with serum hepatitis, or carriers of the serum hepatitis virus, have been found to harbor an antigen in their bloodstream which can be demonstrated by specialized laboratory tests. The antigen is called *Australia antigen* (because it was first discovered in the blood of an Australian native). It is also called *hepatitis-associated antigen* (HAA). The exact nature of this antigen is uncertain, but it appears likely that it represents a fragment of the hepatitis virus. Recognition of carriers of the serum hepatitis virus is important, since a person whose blood contains the virus should not be used as a blood donor. Therefore, many blood banks screen the blood of donors for the presence of Australia antigen, and those in whom the antigen is demonstrated are considered unsuitable for blood donation. HAA is *not* found in association with the infectious hepatitis virus.

PREVENTION AND TREATMENT OF VIRAL HEPATITIS

If a person has been exposed to hepatitis, the administration of gamma globulin provides some protection against infectious hepatitis, but it is ineffective in preventing serum hepatitis. No specific treatment exists for hepatitis other than bed rest and various supportive measures. The blood and excreta of patients with viral hepatitis should be considered infectious, and nursing personnel caring for patients with hepatitis should use caution to avoid becoming infected. The patient with serum hepatitis may be less infectious than the patient with infectious hepatitis. However, diligence should be used when caring for patients with both types of viral hepatitis.

Fatty Liver

Fatty liver is a special type of liver injury in which fat accumulates in liver cells. A number of injurious agents are capable of disrupting the metabolic processes within the liver cell, leading to such accumulation of fat. In this country, the most common cause of fatty liver is excessive alcohol ingestion. Fatty liver is relatively common in heavy drinkers and in persons who are chronic alcoholics. In addition to alcohol, a number of volatile solvents, drugs, chemicals, and some poisons can cause a fatty liver. Heavy fat infiltration impairs liver function, and prolonged fatty infiltration may eventually cause liver scarring.

Cirrhosis

Cirrhosis of the liver refers to diffuse scarring of the liver from any cause. Any substance capable of injuring the liver may cause cirrhosis under certain conditions. The following are the more common causes of cirrhosis: (1) prolonged fatty infiltration (most common in heavy drinkers), (2) an episode of severe liver necrosis, as after a bout of severe viral hepatitis (sometimes called *posthepatic cirrhosis* or *postnecrotic cirrhosis*), and (3) repeated episodes of liver injury from various causes, or chronic progressive damage to liver cells. In this country, most cases of cirrhosis are related to heavy alcohol ingestion. Other cases follow viral hepatitis or liver injury due to various drugs and chemicals. Often, the actual cause of cirrhosis in a given patient cannot be determined.

In cirrhosis, the liver is converted into a mass of scar tissue containing nodules of degenerating and of regenerating liver cells, proliferating bile ducts, and inflammatory cells. The normal architectural pattern of the liver is completely disorganized, and the intrahepatic branches of the hepatic artery and portal vein are constricted by scar tissue.

The two major functional disturbances in cirrhosis are impaired liver function and portal hypertension.

IMPAIRED LIVER FUNCTION

As a result of liver cell damage, scarring, and impairment of blood supply to the liver due to scarring, the number of functioning liver cells is markedly reduced. Eventually the patient with cirrhosis may die of liver failure.

PORTAL HYPERTENSION

Normally, the portal vein blood passes through sinusoids into the hepatic veins and then into the inferior vena cava. In cirrhosis, venous return through the portal system is impaired, and the pressure in the portal vein rises because of obstruction to the blood flow due to scar tissue. The high pressure is reflected in the portal capillaries, and this contributes to excessive leakage of fluid from the capillaries. Eventually the abdomen becomes distended because of accumulation of fluid within the abdominal cavity. This is called *ascites*.

Because of the obstruction of portal venous return, collateral channels develop which attempt to bypass the block within the liver and deliver blood directly into the vena cava. One route consists of the collateral veins over the abdominal wall, which empty either via the intercostal and internal mammary veins into the superior vena cava, or into the iliac veins and then into the inferior vena cava. Another collateral channel is the veins around the stomach connecting with the esophageal veins, and then into the vena cava. The veins are not equipped to handle the increased blood flow and high pressure and become dilated. The dilated veins in the distal esophagus are called *esophageal varices*. These veins may rupture, leading to massive and often fatal hemorrhage.

Cholelithiasis

Occasionally, cholesterol and pigment from the bile may precipitate, forming gallstones. This condition is called *cholelithiasis* (*chole* = bile + *lith* = stone). Why some individuals develop gallstones and others do not remains unknown. In some cases, infection of the gallbladder predisposes to stone formation. However, most patients with gallstones do not have cholecystitis. Gallstones cause no symptoms as long as they remain in the gallbladder. However, a small stone may be squeezed out of the gallbladder and become impacted in the biliary duct system, causing severe, cramp-like pain, called *biliary colic*. If the stone becomes lodged in the common bile duct, the outflow of bile into the duodenum is blocked and the affected individual becomes jaundiced. If the stone becomes impacted in the cystic duct, the individual may experience considerable pain but will not become jaundiced because the common bile duct remains patent.

Cholecystitis

Cholecystitis refers to inflammation of the gallbladder and is a relatively common disease. Chronic cholecystitis appears to predispose an individual to the development of gallstones.

Tumors

Primary tumors of the liver and gallbladder are uncommon. However, the liver is a frequent site of metastatic carcinoma. Carcinoma arising in the gastrointestinal tract may spread to the liver, bits of tumor being carried in the portal venous blood to lodge in the liver. Tumors from lung, breast, and other sites may also spread to the liver, the tumor being carried in the blood delivered to the liver by the hepatic artery. Sometimes, enlargement of the liver due to metastatic carcinoma may be the first sign of a malignant tumor which originated in some other part of the body.

Jaundice

Jaundice indicates that bile pigments are being retained within the circulation; this can be due to several causes. As previously discussed, bile pigment is derived from the breakdown of red cells. The pigment is extracted from the blood by the liver cells, conjugated, and excreted into the biliary ducts (Fig. 24-2). It is convenient to classify jaundice on the basis of the disturbance responsible for the retention of bile pigment. On this basis, jaundice is classified as *hemolytic, hepatocellular,* or *obstructive.* Proper classification of jaundice can usually be made on the basis of certain laboratory tests in conjunction with the clinical features.

HEMOLYTIC JAUNDICE

In conditions associated with accelerated breakdown of red cells, excessive bile pigment is delivered to the liver, beyond the liver's ability to conjugate and excrete the pigment. Therefore, unconjugated bile pigment accumulates in the blood. Hemolytic jaundice is sometimes seen in adults with hemolytic anemia, but it is encountered most frequently in newborn infants with hemolytic disease due to blood group incompatibility between mother and infant (Chapter 21).

HEPATOCELLULAR JAUNDICE

If the liver is severely damaged, as in hepatitis or cirrhosis, conjugation of bilirubin is impaired. Moreover, the excretion of conjugated bilirubin is profoundly hampered because of injury to liver cells and disruption of small bile channels which lie between liver cell cords. As a result, conjugated bilirubin leaks back into the blood because of the rupture of small bile channels within the liver.

OBSTRUCTIVE JAUNDICE

In obstructive jaundice, the extraction and conjugation of bilirubin by liver cells are not impaired, but jaundice develops because the bile duct is obstructed, preventing delivery of bile into the duodenum. Often this is due to an impacted stone in the common duct. Carcinoma of the head of the pancreas is another common cause of common bile duct obstruction. As indicated in Figure 24-1, the common duct passes very close to the head of the pancreas as it enters the duodenum. Therefore, a pancreatic tumor frequently compresses and invades the common duct.

Liver Biopsy

Many times the exact cause and extent of liver disease is difficult to determine in a given patient. In such cases, a biopsy of the liver can be performed by inserting a needle through the skin directly into the liver and extracting a small bit of liver tissue. This can be examined microscopically by the pathologist, and generally an exact diagnosis can be made concerning the nature and severity of the liver disease. This information can provide a basis for proper treatment.

Chapter 25

The Pancreas

THE PANCREAS consists of two parts. The major portion is concerned with the production of digestive enzymes, discharged through the pancreatic duct into the duodenum. The second part consists of multiple small clusters of highly specialized cells which produce insulin, the *pancreatic islets* or *islets of Langerhans*.

Tumors of the Pancreas

Carcinoma of the pancreas is relatively common, occurring most often in the head of the pancreas. In this location, the neoplasm blocks the common bile duct, resulting in obstructive jaundice. Carcinoma elsewhere in the pancreas is usually far advanced when first detected and produces no specific symptoms.

Occasionally, insulin-secreting tumors arise from the pancreatic islets. The tumors produce symptoms similar to those induced by an overdosage of insulin.

Pancreatitis

ACUTE PANCREATITIS

Acute pancreatitis is due to escape of pancreatic juice from the ducts into the substance of the pancreas. This causes widespread destruction of pancreatic tissue and marked hemorrhage, resulting from the action of the pancreatic digestive enzymes. Patients with acute pancreatitis have severe abdominal pain and are seriously ill; the disease is associated with a high mortality.

The basic cause of acute pancreatitis appears to be active secretion of pancreatic juice in the presence of obstruction of the pancreatic duct at its entrance into the duodenum. These factors markedly increase the pressure within the duct system, causing rupture of ducts and escape of pancreatic juice. Two factors predispose to acute pancreatitis: disease of the gallbladder and excessive alcohol consumption.

Patients with gallstones may develop pancreatitis, because the common bile duct and common pancreatic duct often enter the duodenum through a common channel (the ampulla of Vater). If a stone becomes impacted in the ampulla, this can obstruct the pancreatic duct and precipitate pancreatitis.

Patients who drink excessive amounts of alcohol are also prone to pancreatitis. Alcohol is a potent stimulus to pancreatic secretion; alcohol may also induce edema and spasm of the pancreatic sphincter in the ampulla of Vater. Pancreatitis develops due to the combination of alcohol-induced hypersecretion in conjunction with sphincter spasm, leading to high intraductal pressure, followed by duct necrosis and escape of pancreatic juice.

Chronic Pancreatitis

Occasionally patients develop repeated episodes of mild inflammation within the pancreas, leading to progressive destruction of pancreatic tissue. This is called chronic pancreatitis.

Diabetes Mellitus

Diabetes is one of the most common and important metabolic diseases. It is primarily a disturbance of carbohydrate metabolism due to inadequate output of insulin by the pancreatic islets.

Actions of Insulin

Insulin is required for efficient utilization of glucose by muscle and adipose tissue. Some tissues, such as nerve tissue and red cells, require no insulin. Insulin appears to act by promoting entry of glucose into the cell; it also promotes conversion of glucose into glycogen by the liver. In addition, insulin exerts indirect effects on both protein and fat metabolism, bringing about protein synthesis in muscle and fat deposition in adipose tissue.

Biochemical Disturbances in Diabetes

In diabetes mellitus, glucose is absorbed normally. However, because of lack of insulin, it is not used normally for energy and is not stored normally as glycogen. Consequently, it accumulates in the bloodstream, resulting in a high level of blood glucose. Because of the high blood

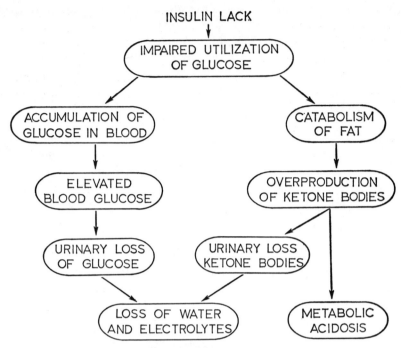

Fig. 25-1.—Major metabolic derangements in diabetes.

glucose, the glucose "spills over" in the urine and is excreted. Since glucose must be excreted in the urine in solution, excessive amounts of water and electrolytes are also lost in the urine. This frequently leads to disturbance in water balance and acid-base balance.

Protein and fat metabolism are also disturbed in diabetes. Protein synthesis is compromised, and body protein is broken down into amino acids. The amino acids are converted to glucose by the liver, augmenting the hyperglycemia and leading to additional losses of glucose, water, and electrolytes in the urine. Fat deposition as adipose tissue is impaired, and body fat is mobilized as a source of energy. Ketone bodies (acetoacetic acid and beta-hydroxybutyric acid), formed as a product of the catabolism of fat, are normally metabolized further to carbon dioxide and water. However, the excessive mobilization of fat as a source of energy leads to formation of large quantities of ketone bodies, which are produced in excess of the body's ability to metabolize them. Ketone bodies accumulate in the blood and "spill over" into the urine. The acid ketone bodies can be buffered to some extent by the bicarbonate buffer system. However, if the diabetes is extremely severe and large amounts of ketone bodies are produced, the buffer systems may be inadequate to maintain normal pH, and *diabetic acidosis* develops. Additional electrolytes and water are lost, associated with excretion of ketone bodies, further complicating the acid-base abnormalities and the disturbances of water balance. All of these effects can be reversed by supplying insulin, which promotes normal utilization of glucose and storage of glycogen. The secondary disturbances in fat and protein metabolism are also reversed by the action of insulin. Figure 25-1 summarizes the major metabolic disturbances in diabetes.

COMPLICATIONS OF DIABETES

Three major complications attend poorly controlled diabetes. The first is an increased susceptibility to infection, apparently related to the high levels of blood sugar. Pathogenic bacteria seem to grow more readily in the presence of elevated blood glucose levels. The second complication is an increased tendency to arteriosclerosis, probably related in part to the abnormalities in fat metabolism and to the elevated blood lipids frequently found in diabetes. The third complication is diabetic coma. This is a severe acidosis associated with marked disturbances in both electrolyte and water balance.

TREATMENT OF DIABETES

Treatment of diabetes consists of a diet in which the carbohydrate intake is limited, often in conjunction with insulin administration (by subcutaneous injection). Oral hypoglycemic drugs are also available, and some diabetics can be managed by these drugs rather than insulin. Mild diabetes can often be controlled by diet alone, without supplementary hypoglycemic agents.

Chapter 26

The Gastrointestinal Tract

THE GASTROINTESTINAL TRACT, which is concerned with the digestion and absorption of food, comprises the oral cavity, esophagus, stomach, small and large intestines, and anus.

Lesions of the Oral Cavity

An inflammation of the oral cavity is called a *stomatitis* (*stoma* = mouth). This may be due to a number of irritants and infectious agents.

Carcinoma of the oral cavity, which may arise from the squamous epithelium of the lips, cheek, tongue, palate, or back of the throat, is relatively common. It is treated by surgical resection or radiation therapy.

Esophageal Obstruction

The esophagus is a muscular tube which conveys food and saliva to the stomach by peristaltic action. Obstruction of the esophagus leads to inability to swallow. This is often associated with regurgitation of food and saliva into the trachea, causing episodes of choking and coughing. Three common causes of obstruction are carcinoma, impaction of food in the esophagus, and stricture.

CARCINOMA OF THE ESOPHAGUS

Carcinoma may arise anywhere in the esophagus, gradually narrowing the lumen. The tumor frequently infiltrates the surrounding tissues and may invade the trachea, leading to the formation of a fistula between trachea and esophagus.

FOOD IMPACTION

Obstruction of the esophagus may be due to impaction of poorly chewed meat in the distal portion of the esophagus. This is sometimes encountered in persons who are unable to chew their food properly because of poor teeth or improperly fitting dentures, or who have poor eating habits.

STRICTURE

A stricture is a narrowing of the esophagus caused by scar tissue. The scarring may result from accidental or deliberate swallowing of a corrosive chemical. This causes necrosis and inflammation of the esophagus, eventually followed by marked scarring. Accidental swallowing of commercial lye solutions by children (used for cleaning clogged drains) is a common cause of esophageal stricture.

Chronic Peptic Ulcer

Peptic ulcer is a chronic ulcer, most commonly involving the distal stomach or proximal duodenum. It is due to digestion of the mucosa by the hydrochloric acid and digestive enzymes in gastric juice.

The factors responsible for the initial peptic ulceration are not completely understood. However, the most important factor appears to be excessive secretion of acid gastric juice. Nervous, high-strung persons and individuals under considerable emotional strain seem to be prone to ulcers. Such individuals also secrete large volumes of extremely acid gastric juice; this is probably the major factor responsible for the high incidence of ulcers in this group.

Probably the initial event is a small, superficial erosion of the gastric or duodenal mucosa. Gastric acid and pepsin begin to digest the deeper tissues which have been denuded of covering epithelium. Attempts at healing in the presence of continuing digestion eventually lead to considerable scarring at the base of the ulcer. Clinically, ulcers produce pain which is usually relieved by ingestion of food or antacids that neutralize the gastric acid.

There are three complications of peptic ulcer: bleeding, perforation, and obstruction. An ulcer which erodes into a large blood vessel may cause severe bleeding. An ulcer may also completely digest the wall of the stomach or duodenum, causing a perforation of the wall. This leads to leakage of gastric and duodenal contents into the peritoneal cavity, resulting in generalized peritonitis. Sometimes such marked scarring follows the healing of a gastric ulcer that the pylorus may be obstructed by scar tissue, preventing proper emptying of the stomach.

In general, peptic ulcer is treated by antacids which neutralize the excess gastric acid and promote healing of the ulcer. Sometimes surgical treatment is required if medical therapy fails to heal the ulcer or if complications develop, such as hemorrhage, perforation, or obstruction.

Carcinoma of the Stomach

At one time, carcinoma of the stomach was the most common malignant tumor in men. Recently, the incidence of gastric carcinoma has been decreasing. The reason for this change is unknown. Gastric carcinoma is treated by resection of a large part of the stomach. Unfortunately, the carcinoma is usually far advanced by the time it causes symptoms, so that long-term survival of patients with stomach carcinoma is relatively poor.

Sometimes gastric carcinoma may produce symptoms similar to those of a benign peptic ulcer. At times it may be difficult for the physician to determine whether a patient has a benign peptic ulcer of the stomach or an ulcerated gastric carcinoma.

Inflammatory Disease of the Intestine

The intestine may be the site of both acute and chronic inflammation. The term *enteritis* (*enteron* = bowel) refers to an inflammation of any portion of the intestinal tract. The term *colitis* denotes inflammation restricted to the colon. Inflammation of the bowel produces symptoms of crampy abdominal pain and diarrhea. If the mucosa of the bowel is ulcerated, blood may appear in the stools.

ACUTE ENTERITIS

Acute enteritis is relatively common and may be caused by many different pathogenic organisms or bacterial toxins. The disease is relatively acute and self-limited.

CHRONIC ENTERITIS

Chronic enteritis is less common than acute enteritis. Two types are recognized: (1) regional enteritis, localized chiefly to the distal ileum, and (2) chronic ulcerative colitis, involving the large intestine. The causes of both types of chronic enteritis are unknown.

REGIONAL ENTERITIS.—Regional enteritis is a chronic inflammation involving primarily the distal ileum. It is characterized by ulceration of the mucosa and marked thickening and scarring of the bowel wall. The inflammation often involves scattered areas of the small bowel, leaving normal intervening areas (called "skip areas") between the areas of severe disease. Treatment usually consists of surgical resection of the involved portion of the bowel.

CHRONIC ULCERATIVE COLITIS.—This is a chronic recurrent inflammation with ulceration of the mucosa of the colon, often involving the entire colon and rectum. Treatment usually consists of surgical resection of the diseased colon.

COMPLICATIONS OF CHRONIC ENTERITIS.—Patients with chronic enteritis often have serious nutritional disturbances due to chronic diarrhea, which leads to poor absorption of food from the diseased bowel. The ulcerated areas in the bowel may bleed profusely. Sometimes the ulcerated areas undergo perforation, leading to leakage of intestinal contents into the peritoneal cavity. Occasionally, patients with regional enteritis have such marked thickening and scarring of the distal small bowel that the lumen becomes blocked, producing signs of intestinal obstruction.

APPENDICITIS

Appendicitis is the most common inflammatory lesion of the bowel. In many animals, the portion of the bowel represented in man by the appendix is a large, wide-caliber intestinal segment, similar in appearance to the remainder of the colon. In man, this segment of bowel is reduced in both size and caliber to the extent that it is a vestigial structure serving no useful function.

The frequency of acute appendicitis is due primarily to the narrow caliber of the appendix, the base of which often becomes plugged by firm bits of fecal material. As a result of the obstruction, there is poor drainage of secretions (normally produced by the epithelial cells lining the appendix) from the area distal to the obstruction. The accumulation of secretions increases intraluminal pressure, which in turn compresses the blood vessels in the mucosa of the appendix, impairing the viability of the appendiceal mucosa. Bacteria normally present in the appendix and colon invade the devitalized wall, causing an acute inflammation. Mild cases of appendicitis may heal spontaneously. More severe inflammation may lead to rupture of the appendix and peritonitis. For this reason, it is common practice to perform an exploratory operation and remove the appendix in any patient in whom appendicitis is suspected.

Diverticulosis and Diverticulitis

Frequently outpouchings of the mucosa of the colon project through weak areas in the muscular wall of the large intestine. These are called *diverticula,* and the condition is called *diverticulosis.* Diverticula are encountered with increasing frequency in older patients; they are located chiefly in the distal portion of the colon. Bits of fecal material may become trapped within these pouches and incite an inflammatory reaction. This is called *diverticulitis*. The inflammation may be followed by considerable scarring. Occasionally, perforation of a diverticulum may occur, leading to an abscess in the pelvis. Sometimes, blood vessels in the mucosa of the diverticulum may become ulcerated due to the trauma of the fecal material, resulting in bleeding. Diverticula attended by such complications as infections or bleeding are often treated by surgical resection of the involved segment of bowel.

Intestinal Obstruction

If the normal passage of intestinal contents through the bowel is blocked, the patient is said to have an intestinal obstruction. The site of the block may be either the small intestine (high intestinal obstruction) or the colon (low intestinal obstruction). Bowel obstruction is always serious. The severity of the symptoms depends on the location of the obstruction, its completeness, and whether there is interference with the blood supply to the blocked segment of bowel.

HIGH INTESTINAL OBSTRUCTION

High intestinal obstruction causes severe, crampy pain due to vigorous peristalsis, reflecting the attempt of the intestine to force bowel contents past the site of obstruction. This is associated with vomiting of copious amounts of gastric and upper intestinal secretions, resulting in loss of large quantities of water and electrolytes. As a consequence, the patient becomes dehydrated and develops pronounced fluid and electrolyte disturbances.

LOW INTESTINAL OBSTRUCTION

Symptoms are much less acute when the distal colon is obstructed. There may be mild crampy abdominal pain and moderate distention of the abdomen. However, vomiting with associated loss of fluid and electrolytes is not as serious a problem as in high intestinal obstruction. Disturbances of fluid and electrolytes do not develop as rapidly.

CAUSES OF INTESTINAL OBSTRUCTION

The common causes of intestinal obstruction are intestinal adhesions, hernia, tumor, volvulus, and intussusception.

Adhesive bands of connective tissue may form within the abdominal cavity after surgery. Sometimes a loop of bowel becomes kinked, compressed, or twisted by an adhesive band, causing obstruction proximal to the site of the adhesion.

A *hernia* is a protrusion of a loop of bowel through a small opening, usually in the abdominal wall. The herniated loop pushes the peritoneum ahead of it, forming the hernia sac. Inguinal hernia is quite common in men. A loop of small bowel protrudes through a weak area in the inguinal ring and may descend downward into the scrotum. Umbilical and femoral hernias occur in both sexes. In an umbilical hernia, the loop of bowel protrudes into the umbilicus through a defect in the abdominal wall. In a femoral hernia, a loop of intestine extends under the inguinal ligament along the course of the femoral vessels into the groin. If a herniated loop of bowel can be pushed back into the abdominal cavity, the hernia is said to be reducible. Occasionally, a herniated loop becomes stuck and cannot be reduced. This is called an *incarcerated hernia.* Sometimes the loop of bowel is so tightly constricted by the margins of the defect which allowed the herniation that the blood supply to the herniated bowel is obstructed, causing necrosis of the protruding segment of bowel. This is called a *strangulated hernia* and requires prompt surgical intervention.

A *volvulus* is a rotary twisting of the bowel on its mesentery, with obstruction of the blood supply to the twisted segment. An intussusception is a telescoping of one segment of bowel into an adjacent segment.

Carcinoma of the colon may obstruct the distal colon and is a common cause of low intestinal obstruction.

Mesenteric Thrombosis

The blood supply to the gastrointestinal tract is derived from several large arteries arising from the aorta. The blood supply to most of the bowel is provided by the superior mesenteric artery. This vessel supplies blood to the entire small intestine and the proximal half of the colon. The arteries supplying the gastrointestinal tract may develop arteriosclerotic changes and become occluded by thrombosis in the same way as other arteries. Thrombosis of the superior mesenteric artery leads to an extensive infarction of most of the bowel, an invariably fatal event.

Carcinoma of the Bowel

Malignant tumors of the small intestine are quite rare, but colon carcinoma is common. Adenocarcinoma may arise anywhere in the colon or rectum. Carcinoma arising in the cecum and right half of the colon generally causes no obstruction of the bowel, since the caliber of this portion of the colon is large, and the bowel contents are relatively soft. However, the tumor often becomes ulcerated and bleeds, leading to chronic iron-deficiency anemia. The patient with a carcinoma of the right half of the colon may consult his physician because of weakness and fatigue due to the anemia, without experiencing any symptoms referable to the intestinal tract.

By contrast, carcinoma of the distal portion of the colon, which has a much smaller caliber, often causes partial obstruction of the bowel and leads to symptoms of lower intestinal obstruction.

Evaluation of Gastrointestinal Disease by the Physician

Unfortunately, most of the gastrointestinal tract cannot be examined as easily as many other parts of the body. However, it is possible to visualize the internal surfaces of both ends of the gastrointestinal tract. This can be accomplished by inserting a long, lighted, tubular instrument into the esophagus or stomach or by inserting a similar type of instrument into the rectum and distal colon. These procedures are frequently performed if the patient experiences symptoms suggesting disease of the esophagus, stomach, or distal colon. Abnormal areas in the mucosa can be visualized, biopsied, and examined histologically.

Areas which cannot be examined directly can be studied by radiologic examination. Examination of the upper gastrointestinal tract is accomplished by having the patient ingest a radiopaque material, after which the physician is able to visualize the transport of the material through the intestinal tract by x-ray studies. He can observe any areas where the motility of the bowel appears abnormal, indicating disease. This technic also allows the physician to visualize the contours of the gastrointestinal mucosa and to thereby identify the location and extent of disease affecting the bowel mucosa, such as ulcer, stricture, tumor, or area of chronic inflammation. The colon can be studied in a similar manner by instilling radiopaque material into the bowel through the anus, in order to outline the contours of the large intestine. This type of study is called a *barium enema.*

Chapter 27

Water, Electrolyte, and Acid-Base Balance

ABOUT 70 per cent of the body consists of water. Most is present within cells as *intracellular water*. The remainder, called *extracellular water*, is present within the interstitial tissues surrounding the cells and in the blood plasma. The body water contains dissolved mineral salts (electrolytes) which dissociate in solution, yielding positively charged ions (cations) and negatively charged ions (anions). The body fluids are electrically neutral, and the sum of the positively charged ions in solution is always balanced by the sum of the negatively charged ions. The concentrations of the individual ions may vary in disease, but electrical neutrality is always maintained.

For purposes of description, it is convenient to consider separately disturbances of body water and abnormalities in the concentrations of electrolytes. However, this separation is artificial, since all body fluids contain dissolved mineral salts. If the electrolyte concentration of the body changes, there is usually a corresponding change in body water. Conversely, changes in body water are usually associated with changes in electrolyte concentrations.

Interrelationships of Intracellular and Extracellular Fluid

Fluid and electrolytes diffuse freely between the intravascular and interstitial fluids. However, the capillaries are impermeable to protein, so that the interstitial fluid contains very little protein.

The fluid within the cells is separated from the interstitial fluid by the cell membrane, which is freely permeable to water but relatively impermeable to sodium and potassium ions. The main extracellular ions are sodium and chloride, whereas the main intracellular ions are potassium and phosphate. The differences in the concentration of the ions on different sides of the cell membrane are due to the metabolic activity of the cell.

In general, the amount of sodium in the body determines the volume of the extracellular fluid, since this is the chief extracellular cation, and the amount of potassium in the body determines the volume of the intracellular fluid, since this is the chief intracellular cation.

Units of Concentration of Electrolytes

In dealing with disturbances of electrolytes, the physician is concerned primarily with concentrations of the various ions and with the interrelationship of positively and negatively charged ions to one another, rather than with the actual number of milligrams or grams of the various salts dissolved in the plasma. Therefore, the concentrations of electrolytes are expressed in units that define their ability to combine with other ions. The quantity which expresses "combining weight" is termed the *equivalent weight*. An equivalent weight is the molecular weight of a substance in grams divided by its valence. When 1 equivalent weight of a substance is dissolved in a solution to make one liter, the concentration is *one equivalent per liter*. In the case of a monovalent substance, this is the same as a molar solution. As an example, the equivalent weight of sodium chloride is 23 (molecular weight of sodium) plus 35.5 (molecular weight of chloride), divided by the valence (which is 1), equals 58.5 grams of sodium chloride, the *equivalent weight*. In body fluids, the concentrations of electrolytes are low and are usually expressed in milliequivalents per liter (abbreviated mEq/L) rather than in equivalents. A milliequivalent is 1/1,000 of an equivalent. Concentrations of ions expressed in milliequivalents have equal combining properties, even though their equivalent weights are not equal. For example, a milliequivalent of bicarbonate ion is equal in electrical and ionic characteristics to a milliequivalent of chloride ion, even though the molecular weight of bicarbonate is greater than that of chloride.

Regulation of Body Fluid and Electrolyte Concentrations

The amount of water and electrolytes in the body represents a balance between the amounts ingested in food and fluids and the amounts excreted in the urine, through the gastrointestinal tract, in perspiration, and as water vapor excreted by the lungs. The kidney is important in controlling the concentration of body water and electrolytes. Under the influence of adrenal cortical and posterior pituitary hormones, the kidneys regulate the internal environment of the body by either selectively excreting or retaining water and electrolytes as required to maintain a uniform composition of the body fluids.

Disturbances of Water Balance

DEHYDRATION

The most common disturbance of water balance is dehydration. This may be due to inadequate water intake or excess loss of water. Most cases of dehydration seen in medical practice result from excessive loss of fluid from the gastrointestinal tract as a consequence of vomiting or diarrhea. Fluid intake is usually also decreased, contributing to the dehydration. Occasionally, comatose or debilitated patients become dehydrated because of inadequate intake of fluid.

OVERHYDRATION

Overhydration is less common than dehydration. Occasionally this results from an excessively large intake of fluids in a patient in whom renal function is impaired. Sometimes overhydration is due to excessive administration of intravenous fluids.

Disturbances of Electrolyte Balance

In general, the same conditions producing disturbances of water balance also disturb the electrolyte composition of the body fluids. Most electrolyte disturbances result from depletion of body electrolytes. Depletion of sodium and potassium generally occur together. Often this is due to loss of electrolytes along with water from the gastrointestinal tract due to vomiting or diarrhea. Large amounts of sodium and potassium may also be lost in the urine as a result of prolonged use of diuretics. Diuretics are substances which promote excretion of salts and water by the kidneys by impairing their reabsorption from the glomerular filtrate; they are often administered to patients with heart failure and certain other diseases. Loss of large amounts of electrolytes may also accompany excessive excretion of water in the urine in uncontrolled diabetes, as a result of the diuretic effect of the excreted glucose (Chapter 25), or due to renal tubular disease, in which the regenerating renal tubules are unable to conserve electrolytes and water (Chapter 22).

Acid-Base Balance

The body may be considered an acid-producing machine generating large amounts of both organic and inorganic acids in consequence of normal metabolic processes. However, the body fluids are slightly alkaline, and the hydrogen ion concentration of the body expressed as pH is held within a very narrow range from about pH 7.38 to 7.42. Control of pH is accomplished by three different systems: the buffer systems of the blood, the lungs, and the kidneys.

BUFFERS

The buffer systems of the blood are the first line of defense against change in pH. In a general sense, a buffer is anything that cushions a blow or absorbs an impact. Chemically, a buffer may be defined as a weak acid and a salt of the acid, or a weak base and its salt. Buffers minimize change in hydrogen ion concentration by converting strong (completely ionized) acids and bases into weaker (less completely dissociated) acids and bases.

The major buffer system of the blood is the *sodium bicarbonate–carbonic acid system.* This system is of major importance because both components of the buffer system are present in large amounts, and the concentration of each component can be regulated by the body. The concentration of carbonic acid (dissolved carbon dioxide) is controlled by the lung, and the concentration of bicarbonate is controlled by the kidney. Although the bicarbonate–carbonic acid buffer system is not the only buffer system of the body, the system is in equilibrium with the other buffer systems. Therefore, measurement of the components of this system provides an over-all evaluation of the acid-base status of the patient.

RESPIRATORY CONTROL OF CARBONIC ACID.—Carbonic acid represents physically dissolved carbon dioxide in plasma. This is in equilibrium with the carbon dioxide in the pulmonary alveoli. (The concentration of a gas is expressed in terms of its *partial pressure;* it is also common to speak of the partial pressure as the *tension* of the gas.) Hyperventilation lowers the alveolar carbon dioxide partial pressure (tension) and leads to a rapid decrease in the concentration of carbon dioxide in the plasma. Decreased or inadequate pulmonary ventilation results in elevation of alveolar carbon dioxide tension, and this is associated with an increase in plasma carbonic acid concentration.

CONTROL OF BICARBONATE CONCENTRATION.—The bicarbonate concentration in the plasma is regulated by the kidneys. This is accomplished by selective reabsorption of filtered bicarbonate as necessary to meet the body's requirements. In addition, the kidneys are capable of manufacturing bicarbonate to replace the amounts lost in buffering acids produced as a consequence of normal metabolic processes.

RELATION BETWEEN pH OF BUFFER AND CONCENTRATION OF COMPONENTS.

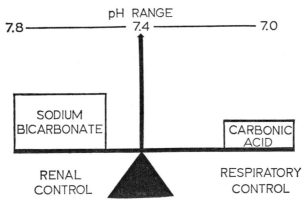

Fig. 27-1.—"Board-and-fulcrum" concept of normal bicarbonate–carbonic acid relationships.

In any buffer system the pH depends upon the ratio of the two components and not upon the absolute quantities of the components. In the case of the bicarbonate–carbonic acid buffer system, at normal body pH of 7.4, the normal ratio consists of 20 parts of sodium bicarbonate and one part of carbonic acid.

Another way of visualizing the bicarbonate–carbonic acid relationship is to think of a board on a fulcrum. One side of the board is weighted by 20 parts of sodium bicarbonate, and the other side is weighted by one part of carbonic acid. The fulcrum is placed so that the board is exactly in balance, corresponding to a body pH of 7.4. Variations in the "weight" of either the sodium bicarbonate or carbonic acid can be visualized as unbalancing the board, resulting in a shift of pH to a new pH, either higher or lower than the normal value (Fig. 27-1).

Disturbances of Acid-Base Balance

Disturbances in which blood pH is shifted to the acid side of the physiologic range is called *acidosis*. This may be due to an excess of carbonic acid or a reduced amount of bicarbonate. A shift in the opposite direction is termed *alkalosis*. This may be due to a decrease in carbon dioxide or an excess of bicarbonate. These possibilities allow classification of acid-base disturbances into four large categories: (1) metabolic acidosis (decrease in bicarbonate), (2) respiratory acidosis (increase in carbonic acid), (3) metabolic alkalosis (increase in bicarbonate), and (4) respiratory alkalosis (decrease in carbonic acid).

The term "metabolic" is applied when the disturbance involves primarily the bicarbonate member of the buffer pair. The term "respiratory" indicates that the primary disturbance lies in the carbonic acid component of the buffer.

COMPENSATORY MECHANISMS FOLLOWING DISTURBANCES IN pH

If the acid-base disturbance shifts the pH outside of the physiologic range, various control measures are activated which attempt to resist the change in pH. This is accomplished by compensatory mechanisms which attempt to preserve the normal 20:1 ratio of bicarbonate to carbonic acid, and thereby return the pH to the physiologic range. For example, if the concentration of carbonic acid rises, there is a compensatory increase in bicarbonate which tends to restore the ratio of the two constituents and maintain pH in the physiologic range. Conversely, if there is a decrease in bicarbonate, compensation involves a decrease in the concentration of carbonic acid in order to maintain a relatively normal ratio. The body's major concern is maintaining a normal ratio of constituents in order to maintain a physiologic pH, even though this is accomplished by changing the absolute concentrations of the members of the buffer pair. Compensation is accomplished by both renal and respiratory methods.

For the student attempting to grasp the fundamentals of the major disturbances in acid-base balance, the "board-and-fulcrum" concept is frequently helpful (Fig. 27-1). The "weight" of carbonic acid is controlled by respiration, and the "weight" of bicarbonate is controlled by renal excretion or conservation of bicarbonate. The student should consider two things: (1) the nature of the primary disturbance and how it will "unbalance" the board, and (2) the steps the body should take to bring the board back into balance. These are the compensatory mechanisms, and they generally consist of "adding weight" or "subtracting weight" from the other member of the board. Admittedly, this is a mechanical oversimplification of a complex process, but it is a helpful learning device when the student is first introduced to the subject.

The two most common clinical disturbances of acid-base balance are metabolic acidosis and respiratory acidosis.

METABOLIC ACIDOSIS

Metabolic acidosis is encountered commonly by the physician. It may be due to impaired renal function, leading to retention of acids generated in normal metabolic processes which would normally be excreted by the kidneys (Chapter 22). Metabolic acidosis may also be due to overproduction of ketone bodies (acetoacetic acid and beta-hydroxybutyric acid) caused by incomplete combustion of fat, as in diabetic acidosis or starva-

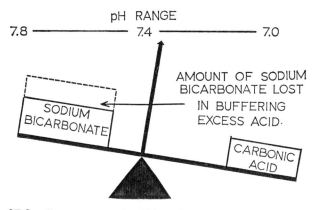

Fig. 27-2.—Derangement of acid-base balance in metabolic acidosis.

tion (Chapter 25). Bicarbonate is reduced because it is consumed in buffering the excess acid (Fig. 27-2). Compensation involves primarily a reduction in carbonic acid. This is accomplished by increasing the rate and depth of respiration, thereby lowering alveolar carbon dioxide tension, which in turn lowers the plasma carbonic acid. Renal compensation is accomplished by reabsorption of as much filtered bicarbonate as possible.

RESPIRATORY ACIDOSIS

In respiratory acidosis, the primary abnormality is failure to excrete carbon dioxide normally. This is usually secondary to chronic lung disease, such as pulmonary emphysema, but it may occur in any situation

Fig. 27-3.—Derangement of acid-base balance in respiratory acidosis.

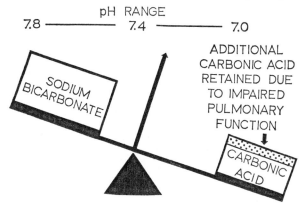

in which pulmonary ventilation is markedly impaired (Chapter 18). In many instances, a respiratory infection in a patient with an underlying chronic lung disease may precipitate acute respiratory acidosis.

Retention of carbon dioxide produces a high alveolar carbon dioxide tension, which in turn leads to an increased plasma carbonic acid, shifting pH to the acid side of the physiologic range (Fig. 27-3). The body's compensatory mechanisms involve conservation of bicarbonate by the kidney, leading to an increase in plasma bicarbonate. This shifts the pH back toward the more physiologic range, since the ratio of the component has been at least partially restored toward normal.

Metabolic Alkalosis

Metabolic alkalosis is less common than the other two disturbances. It is most often caused by loss of chloride. Chloride and bicarbonate are the major negative ions in the plasma, and their concentrations are interrelated. Loss of chloride, as from excessive vomiting, is associated with compensatory elevation in bicarbonate to maintain a normal concentration of negatively charged ions. In most instances, loss of chloride is also associated with potassium depletion, since the body has a limited ability to conserve potassium. Compensatory measures in metabolic alkalosis are relatively ineffective. Decreased alveolar ventilation tends to elevate alveolar carbon dioxide tension and lead to elevation of carbonic acid in the plasma. But this compensation is quite limited, since adequate ventilation is required to produce adequate oxygenation of the blood. Renal compensation occurs by increased excretion of bicarbonate. However, the potassium-deficient kidney functions inefficiently, and therefore renal compensation is relatively ineffective in the presence of potassium depletion.

Respiratory Alkalosis

The basic abnormality is a reduction in the carbonic acid component of the buffer pair. This is due to *hyperventilation*, either because of stimulation of the respiratory center by drugs, certain types of neurologic disease, or occasionally emotional disturbances. The result of hyperventilation is a relative excess of bicarbonate relative to the reduced carbonic acid, so that the normal ratio is no longer maintained. Compensation is primarily by renal excretion of bicarbonate, thereby reducing the concentration of bicarbonate in the plasma and restoring the ratio of components toward normal.

EVALUATION OF ACID-BASE BALANCE BY THE PHYSICIAN

In evaluating the acid-base status of a patient, the physician frequently determines the concentration of the bicarbonate in the plasma as an index of the individual's over-all status. This is supplemented in many cases by the determination of the blood pH and the determination of the carbonic acid in the plasma. The clinical state of the patient, as evaluated by the physician, together with these various laboratory tests, generally permits a determination of the patient's acid-base status and serves as a guide for effective treatment.

Chapter 28

Endocrine Glands

ENDOCRINE GLANDS liberate their secretions directly into the bloodstream, exerting a regulatory effect on various metabolic functions. The major endocrine glands are the pituitary, thyroid, parathyroids, adrenal cortex and medulla, pancreatic islets, ovaries, and testes. In addition to these glands, certain other specialized cells elaborate secretions with an endocrine function, but by convention these are not generally considered in a discussion of the endocrine system.

A disorder of an endocrine gland may consist of either hypersecretion of the gland, reflected as overactivity of the target organ regulated by the gland, or insufficient secretion, resulting in underactivity of the organ controlled by the gland.

The clinical effects of a disturbance of endocrine gland function are determined by the degree of dysfunction of the gland and the age and sex of the affected individual. All degrees of glandular dysfunction may be encountered, ranging from barely detectable variations from normal to profound degrees of hypofunction or hyperfunction. The age of the person when the endocrine disturbance becomes manifest has a pronounced effect on the clinical features. Some endocrine glands, such as the thyroid gland, affect growth and development as well as metabolic processes, so that disturbed function in the child will produce a somewhat different clinical picture than a similar disturbance in the adult. The sex of the individual also influences the effect of disturbed endocrine function. Many hormones are concerned with the development and maintenance of sexual function and secondary sexual characteristics, and several endocrine glands elaborate sex hormones. Some endocrine disturbances cause alteration in sexual development in a child, whereas the effects are much less pronounced in the adult. Overproduction of an inappropriate sex hormone in some endocrine diseases causes masculinization of the female or feminization of the male; on the other hand, overproduction of a sex hormone appropriate to the sex of the individual has little clinical effect.

Pituitary Gland

The pituitary gland has often been called "the master gland of the body" because it exerts a regulatory influence on most of the endocrine glands. It is composed of an anterior lobe, a posterior lobe, and a small intermediate lobe. Elaboration of the various hormones of the anterior lobe is regulated by humoral substances called *releasing factors*. These are synthesized in the hypothalamus and transmitted to the anterior lobe by a system of portal blood vessels which establish vascular connection between the hypothalamus and the pituitary gland. The posterior lobe hormones are synthesized within the hypothalamus and are transmitted to the posterior lobe along nerve fibers for storage in the posterior lobe. Release of neural secretions from the posterior lobe is accomplished by nerve impulses transmitted to the posterior lobe from the hypothalamus. The hypothalamus, in turn, is under the control of higher cortical centers, so that the pituitary secretion is to some extent indirectly influenced by external stimuli conveyed to the nervous system, as well as by mental and emotional stimuli arising in higher cortical centers.

The anterior lobe of the pituitary produces growth hormone, thyroid-stimulating hormone (TSH), adrenocorticotrophic hormone (ACTH), gonadotrophic hormones, and prolactin. The intermediate lobe produces a hormone concerned with skin pigmentation. The posterior lobe produces antidiuretic hormone (ADH) and oxytocin. The functions of these are described briefly below.

Growth hormone, produced by the anterior lobe, has multiple actions, all concerned with general tissue growth. *Thyroid-stimulating hormone (TSH)* stimulates the growth of the thyroid and the production of thyroid hormones. *Adrenocorticotrophic hormone (ACTH)* stimulates the adrenal cortex to manufacture and secrete adrenal cortical steroid hormones. *Gonadotrophic hormones* are responsible for growth and development of the gonads and the development of sexual characteristics related to gonadal function. They help establish and maintain the normal menstrual cycle in the female. Sexual activity and sexual growth and development are impaired in the absence of gonadotrophic hormones. *Prolactin* is concerned chiefly with initiating and maintaining lactation, in conjunction with other hormones; it is also required for the maintenance of the corpus luteum.

Antidiuretic hormone (ADH), produced by the posterior lobe, is concerned with regulation of water balance by influencing the reabsorption of water from the distal portion of the renal tubules. In the absence of ADH, the individual is unable to conserve water and excretes large volumes of dilute urine. *Oxytoxin* stimulates uterine contraction during labor and is concerned with release of the milk from the breast during lactation.

PHYSIOLOGIC CONTROL OF PITUITARY HORMONE SECRETION

The level of the various trophic hormones elaborated by the pituitary is regulated by the level of circulating hormone produced by the target gland (Fig. 28-1). Cells in the hypothalamus measure the level of the various hormones in the blood. When the concentration of hormone falls below a certain level, *releasing factors* are elaborated which travel by the portal venous system to the pituitary gland, causing release of the trophic hormone. This, in turn, affects the target organ. The level of the hormone elaborated by the target organ rises, until it reaches the upper range of normal. At this point, the high level of circulating hormone "shuts off" further elaboration of trophic hormone. This mechanism permits a relatively steady hormone output from the target organ and prevents large fluctuations in hormonal level which would adversely affect metabolic activity.

Fig. 28-1.—Normal mechanisms controlling elaboration of trophic hormones by the pituitary gland.

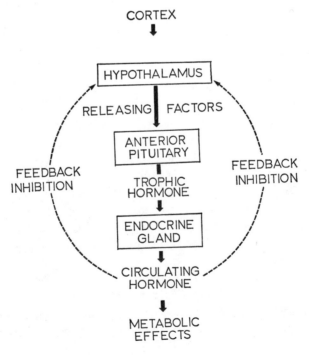

Abnormalities of Pituitary Hormone Secretion

Abnormalities in the secretion of trophic hormones from the pituitary may involve either single or multiple hormones. Isolated deficiencies of single hormones are unusual. Decrease in the secretion of all pituitary hormones, called *panhypopituitarism,* is also uncommon, but occasionally may result from destruction of the pituitary by tumor or disease. Sometimes necrosis of the maternal pituitary gland occurs following childbirth.

Normal growth depends on secretion of adequate amounts of growth hormone by the pituitary. Impaired secretion leads to marked retardation of growth, and usually incomplete sexual development, as well. This is called *pituitary dwarfism.* Administration of growth hormone results in normal growth and development.

Overproduction of growth hormone is usually due to a hormone-secreting tumor of the pituitary gland. The clinical syndrome depends on the age of the patient at the time the tumor appears. Overproduction of growth hormone in children or adolescents, before closure of the epiphyses, causes excessive growth in the length of bones, called *pituitary gigantism.* Some associated coarsening of the facial features also tends to be evident, due to the effect of growth hormone on the structure of the facial bones. Many of the giants seen in circuses are examples of pituitary gigantism. In the adult, excessive production of growth hormone causes *acromegaly.* Since the epiphyses have fused, there can be no growth in height. However, the growth hormone produces thickening and coarsening of bones and generalized enlargement of the viscera. Affected individuals have coarse facial features, large prominent jaws, and large, spadelike hands, but they are no taller than normal. The term acromegaly (*acron* = extremity + *megas* = large) describes one prominent feature of the disease.

Thyroid Gland

The thyroid gland lies in the neck surrounding the trachea. The gland is regulated by pituitary TSH. The level of circulating thyroid hormone, in turn, controls the output of TSH, providing a relatively uniform level of circulating thyroid hormone (Fig. 28-1). The gland has the capacity to extract iodine from the plasma and convert it enzymatically to thyroid hormone. The hormone is stored in the gland and released into the bloodstream as required.

Actions of Thyroid Hormone

Thyroid hormone controls the rate of metabolic processes; it is also required for normal growth and development. An excess of thyroid hor-

TABLE 28-1.—COMPARISON OF MAJOR EFFECTS OF HYPERTHYROIDISM
AND HYPOTHYROIDISM

	HYPERTHYROIDISM	HYPOTHYROIDISM
Cardiovascular effects	Rapid pulse, increased cardiac output	Slow pulse, reduced cardiac output
Metabolic effects	Increased metabolism, skin hot and flushed, weight loss	Decreased metabolism, skin cold, weight gain
Neuromuscular effects	Tremor, hyperactive reflexes	Weakness, lassitude, sluggish reflexes
Mental, emotional effects	Restlessness, irritability, emotional lability	Mental processes sluggish and retarded, personality placid and phlegmatic
Gastrointestinal effects	Diarrhea	Constipation
General somatic effects	Skin warm, moist	Skin cold, dry

mone accelerates all bodily metabolic functions. Conversely, a decrease in the level of thyroid hormone slows metabolic processes. Clinically, some of the most pronounced effects of excess thyroid hormone are reflected in the cardiovascular and neuromuscular systems. The heart rate is accelerated. Reflexes are hyperactive, and frequently a fine tremor of the muscles is apparent. Effects of hormone on emotional and intellectual functions are also conspicuous. Individuals with excess thyroid hormone are hyperactive, emotionally labile, and often quite irritable. They may have difficulty concentrating because mental processes are accelerated excessively. The effects of thyroid hypofunction are the reverse of those in hyperthyroidism. The hypothyroid individual is slow and lethargic. Bodily metabolic functions are subnormal. Reflexes and speech are slow and sluggish. Table 28-1 summarizes the major clinical effects resulting from abnormal levels of thyroid hormone.

ABNORMALITIES OF THYROID FUNCTION

HYPERTHYROIDISM.—Hyperthyroidism in the adult is usually due to a diffuse hyperplasia (enlargement) of the thyroid gland resulting from excessive stimulation by pituitary TSH. The term *goiter* refers to any enlargement of the thyroid gland. Therefore, the hyperactive, enlarged gland is called a *diffuse toxic goiter,* the term "toxic" referring to the injurious hypermetabolic effects of increased thyroid hormone. Another commonly used term is *thyrotoxicosis,* literally meaning "conditions of thyroid toxicity." A third term for diffuse hyperplasia with hyperthyroidism is *Graves' disease.* Hyperthyroid individuals often have prominent, protruding eyes, which gave rise to the term *exophthalmic goiter* (*exo* = out + *ophthalmos* = eye), sometimes applied to this disease.

HYPOTHYROIDISM.—Hypothyroidism in the adult is called *myxedema*. This term is used because the skin of the hypothyroid patient has a puffy appearance due to accumulations of mucinous material in the skin ("myx" refers to mucin). The baggy-eyed look of myxedematous patients is partly related to the mucinous material in the skin around the eyes.

Cretinism is hypothyroidism in the infant. Thyroid hormone is required for normal growth and development and plays an important role in the maturation and development of the nervous system. The cretin manifests the same features as the hypothyroid adult, and in addition is short and mentally retarded. If cretinism is recognized in the neonatal period and treated effectively by administration of thyroid hormone, both mental and physical development will be normal. If not, physical and mental development becomes permanently impaired.

Cretinism may be due to failure of development of the thyroid gland, called *athyreotic cretinism* (*a* = without + thyroid), or to genetically determined deficiencies of enzymes necessary for thyroid hormone synthesis, called *goiterous cretinism*. In the latter, the gland undergoes hyperplasia due to excessive TSH stimulation, but it is incapable of producing adequate hormone because of a congenital deficiency of enzymes in the gland.

GOITER

A goiter is any enlargement of the thyroid gland, whether or not secretion of thyroid hormone is increased. Thyroid enlargement associated with increased output of hormone causes hyperthyroidism and is called *toxic goiter* (already discussed).

A nontoxic goiter is an enlargement of the gland without increased thyroid secretion. The enlargement of the gland may be either diffuse or nodular. Both nodular and diffuse goiters are produced by the same factors. The underlying defect is inadequate output of thyroid hormone, due to any one of three basic causes: (1) iodine deficiency, (2) interference with synthesis of hormone by the thyroid gland, and (3) increased demand for thyroid hormone.

IODINE DEFICIENCY.—If iodine is deficient in the diet, not enough will be available to produce adequate hormone for the needs of the individual. This is an uncommon cause of goiter in this country.

INTERFERENCE WITH SYNTHESIS OF HORMONE BY THE THYROID GLAND.— Conversion of iodine to thyroid hormone involves a number of steps requiring several different enzymes. An individual may have relatively mild congenital deficiencies of certain hormones necessary for hormone synthesis. Or, certain drugs may block some step in hormone synthesis. Moreover, some foods, such as cabbage, turnips, and rutabaga, contain substances (called "goiterogenic substances") which interfere with hormone synthesis by the thyroid, although usually these foods are not eaten in large enough quantities to cause difficulty.

INCREASED DEMAND FOR THYROID HORMONE.—In some persons, iodine intake may be adequate for normal needs, but it may be insufficient when there is an increased requirement for thyroid hormone, as in puberty and pregnancy and under conditions of stress. In these situations, output of hormone is inadequate because of the increased need for hormone.

EFFECT OF DECREASED HORMONE OUTPUT.—When output of thyroid hormone is deficient due to any of these causes, the pituitary responds by an increased output of TSH. This, in turn, leads to enlargement of the thyroid gland. Because of the enlargement of the gland, the thyroid is able to extract iodine more efficiently from the serum and produce a relatively normal output of hormone. However, this occurs at the expense of an increase in the size of the gland (Fig. 28-2). When the increased require-

Fig. 28-2.—Pathogenesis of nontoxic goiter.

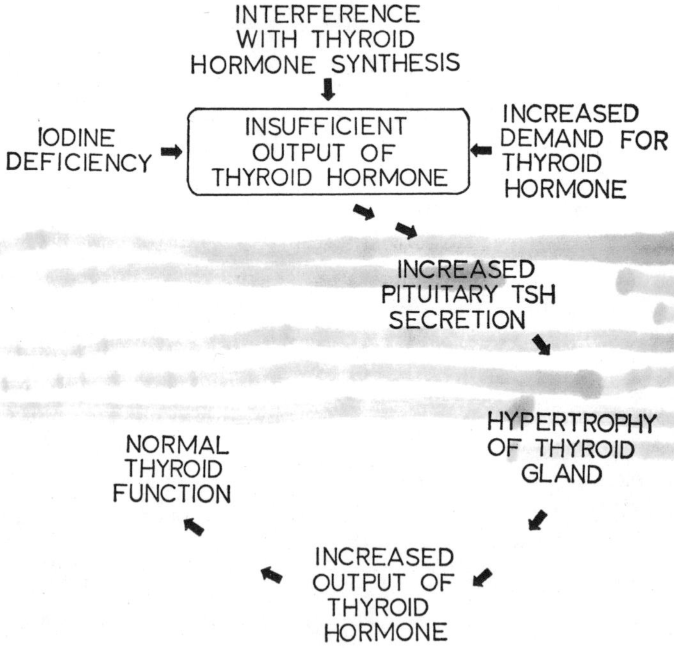

ments of thyroid hormones have been met, or when iodine supplies become available after a period of iodine deficiency, the gland may decrease in size (involution). However, the condition which led to enlargement of the gland often recurs, and the gland undergoes another period of hyperplasia, later followed by involution. Repeated episodes of hyperplasia followed by involution lead to marked variation in the response of the thyroid gland to TSH, eventually causing the development of hyperplastic, tumor-like nodules throughout the gland. This is called *nodular goiter.*

Usually, nodular goiter is treated by administration of thyroid hormone; this suppresses pituitary TSH stimulation of the thyroid gland. The treatment prevents further enlargement of the gland and often causes it to decrease in size. Large, nodular glands may compress the trachea, leading to respiratory distress. Occasionally, markedly enlarged glands require surgical removal.

THYROIDITIS

For reasons that are not well understood, some individuals develop autoantibodies to their own thyroid tissue. The antibodies cause destruction of the thyroid, often leading to hypothyroidism. This disease is generally called *chronic thyroiditis,* and the involved gland is usually enlarged due to a diffuse infiltration by lymphocytes and plasma cells. However, the cellular infiltration is not due to an infection; it is a manifestation of the immunologic reaction between the antigen (thyroid tissue) and the antithyroid antibody. The cellular reaction represents cell-mediated and humoral immune defense reactions (Chapter 4).

Adrenals

The adrenals are paired glands which lie above the kidneys. Each adrenal consists of two separate endocrine organs, the *medulla* and the *cortex.* The medulla secretes adrenalin. Rarely, adrenal medullary tumors arise which elaborate large amounts of this hormone. The adrenal cortex secretes three major classes of steroid hormones: (1) glucocorticoids, (2) mineralocorticoids, and (3) sex hormones.

Glucocorticoids are concerned with regulation of carbohydrate metabolism; they also have an indirect effect on protein metabolism and an anti-inflammatory effect. The major glucocorticoid is *cortisol* (also called *hydrocortisone*). Overproduction of glucocorticoids elevates the level of blood sugar and inhibits the normal inflammatory response. The use of adrenal corticosteroids to treat various types of inflammatory diseases is related to the anti-inflammatory property of the glucocorticoids.

Mineralocorticoids regulate electrolyte and water balance. The major mineralocorticoid is *aldosterone.* Increased aldosterone secretion leads to retention of sodium and water. In contrast to most of the other adrenal steroids, the level of aldosterone is controlled chiefly by the rate of blood flow to the kidney. If the renal blood flow is decreased, specialized cells in the kidney produce a hormonal secretion which indirectly leads to increased aldosterone secretion. One can visualize the kidney as "interpreting" the reduced blood flow to mean that blood volume is low; aldosterone secretion is then called for in order to promote retention of sodium and water, thereby increasing blood volume.

Small amounts of *progesterone, estrogen,* and *androgens* are manufactured in the adrenal glands of both males and females. These probably serve little function under normal circumstances, but in certain diseases there may be overproduction of one or more of these hormones.

ABNORMALITIES OF ADRENAL CORTICAL FUNCTION

Abnormal adrenal cortical function produces abnormalities in the metabolism of carbohydrates and protein due to abnormal glucocorticoid secretion, as well as disturbances of salt and water metabolism due to disturbed mineralocorticoid secretion.

ADDISON'S DISEASE.—Addison's disease is due to atrophy or destruction of the adrenal gland, leading to a deficiency in both glucocorticoids and mineralocorticoids. The patient with Addison's disease has an impaired ability to regulate sodium and water balance and evidence of disturbed carbohydrate metabolism. Because of the reduced output of cortical hormones, ACTH secretion rises; this has an effect on skin pigmentation, resulting in darkening of the skin. Treatment of Addison's disease consists of administration of the deficient corticosteroids.

CUSHING'S DISEASE.—Excessive adrenal corticosteroid production causes Cushing's disease, which may be due to either adrenal hyperplasia or an adrenal tumor. Increased glucocorticoids cause an increased deposition of body fat largely restricted to the trunk, a characteristic "moon" face, elevated blood sugar, and other manifestations of abnormal carbohydrate metabolism. The increased output of mineralocorticoids leads to retention of salt and water; this, in turn, causes an increased blood volume and elevated blood pressure.

Cushing's disease may also be induced by administration of large amounts of adrenal corticosteroid hormones, as in the treatment of leukemia and certain types of collagen diseases.

Cushing's disease due to adrenal hyperplasia or tumor can be cured by surgical removal of the hyperplastic glands or the adrenal neoplasm. Cushing's disease induced by therapeutic administration of steroid hormones can be "cured" by stopping the treatment.

OVERPRODUCTION OF ADRENAL SEX HORMONES.—Adrenal gland dysfunction associated with abnormal production of sex hormone is uncommon. This may result either from *congenital hyperplasia* of the adrenal gland or from an adrenal *sex-hormone-producing tumor.*

Congenital adrenal hyperplasia represents a congenital deficiency of certain enzymes required for the synthesis of various steroid hormones. In the normal biosynthesis of hormones by the adrenal cortex, cholesterol is initially converted to an intermediate compound (pregnenolone) which is a precursor of the other steroids produced in the adrenal (Fig. 28-3). The chief metabolic pathways are concerned with the conversion of the intermediate compound to aldosterone, the major mineralocorticoid (pathway I), and to the glucocorticoid cortisol (pathway II). A third minor metabolic pathway leads to the production of adrenal androgens (pathway III). The biosynthesis of hormones in the major pathways I and II require a series of additions of hydroxyl groups to the steroid molecules, and the enzymes which catalyze these reactions are called *hydroxylases.* If certain hydroxylases are absent or deficient, synthesis of aldosterone and cortisol will be impaired. This leads to increased ACTH secretion (because the pituitary interprets the low steroid levels in the blood as an indication to produce more ACTH). ACTH stimulation produces hyperplasia of the adrenal glands and increased synthesis of precursor com-

Fig. 28-3.—Biosynthesis of adrenal cortical hormones, illustrating site of enzymatic block leading to overproduction of adrenal androgens.

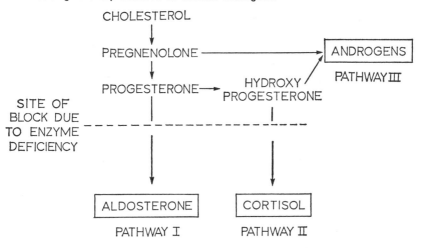

pounds. However, because of the enzymatic block affecting the major pathways of steroid production, biosynthesis is shifted in the direction of androgenic steroids (pathway III). Consequently, the major steroid output from the adrenals consists of androgenic compounds.

The clinical disorder produced by these enzymatic defects is often called the *adrenogenital syndrome*. There are several clinical varieties of this syndrome, depending on which of the hydroxylase enzymes is deficient and the extent of the deficiency. All have the common feature of producing premature sexual development, called *precocious puberty*. In the female, sexual development is masculine because of the effect of the androgens. The age at which the hormonal effects become manifest depends on the degree of the enzyme deficiency. Congenital virilization may be noted at birth. If the deficiency is less severe, symptoms may not appear until the child is older.

Adrenal tumors which elaborate sex hormones are rare. When such a tumor develops, however, either androgen or estrogen may be produced. The clinical features depend on the age of the individual when the tumor becomes manifest and the sex of the affected person. In a child, the tumor produces precocious puberty, and the character of the sexual development depends on the type of hormone elaborated. In the adult, an estrogen-producing neoplasm elicits no hormonal symptoms in the female but induces feminization in the male. An androgen-secreting tumor masculinizes a woman but causes no hormonal symptoms in a man.

Parathyroid Glands

Four very small parathyroid glands lie embedded in the posterior surface of the thyroid gland. The parathyroid hormone regulates the level of calcium in the blood by regulating the release of calcium from bone, the absorption of calcium from the intestine, and the rate of excretion of calcium by the kidneys. In contrast to most other endocrine glands, the secretion of parathyroid hormone is regulated by the level of calcium in the blood, rather than by means of a trophic hormone elaborated by the pituitary gland. If the level of calcium in the blood decreases, the parathyroids make more hormone. If the calcium level rises, parathyroid hormone secretion declines.

ABNORMALITIES OF PARATHYROID FUNCTION

Hyperfunction is the most common disorder of the parathyroid gland, usually due to a benign tumor which secretes excessive amounts of hormone. As a consequence, the level of calcium in the blood rises. Calcium is withdrawn from bone, demineralizing and weakening it. Excessive amounts of calcium are excreted in the urine, sometimes leading to formation of calcium stones within the urinary tract. Occasionally, calcium precipitates out of the blood and becomes deposited in the kidneys, lungs, and other tissues, producing injury and functional impairment. Treatment consists of surgical removal of the tumor.

Hypofunction of parathyroid glands is usually secondary to accidental removal of the parathyroid glands in the course of a surgical operation on the thyroid gland. One method of treatment of hyperthyroidism is surgical removal of most of the thyroid gland; occasionally the parathyroid glands are also removed inadvertently. When this happens, the level of blood calcium drops precipitously. Since calcium is concerned with nerve impulse conduction, low blood calcium results in marked neuromuscular irritability and often muscular spasms called *tetany*.

Pancreas

In addition to manufacturing digestive enzymes, the pancreas functions as an endocrine gland. The specialized cell clusters, the *pancreatic islets*, produce insulin, a hormone concerned with regulating the level of blood glucose. Secretion of insulin is regulated by the level of blood glucose and is not under the control of the pituitary gland. The most common dysfunction of the endocrine portion of the pancreas is diabetes mellitus, which may be considered as a manifestation of decreased function of the pancreatic islets (discussed previously).

Benign tumors of the pancreatic islets occasionally arise in the pancreas and produce symptoms due to excessive secretion of insulin.

Gonads

The gonads have two functions: (1) the production of germ cells, either eggs or sperm, and (2) the production of sex hormones, responsible for the development of secondary sexual characteristics. The latter function is controlled by the gonadotrophic hormones of the pituitary gland. Occasionally sex-hormone-secreting tumors develop in the ovary or testis. They may secrete sex hormone appropriate to the sex of the individual or, paradoxically, sex hormone characteristic of the opposite sex. No endocrine symptoms result from a tumor which produces the "proper" sex hormone; however, elaboration of the inappropriate sex hormone by the tumor causes masculinization in the female or feminization in the male. Sex-hormone-secreting tumors of the gonads are usually benign, and the disorder can be cured by surgical excision.

Obesity

CAUSES OF OBESITY

Fat is the storage form of energy. Any caloric intake which exceeds requirements is stored as adipose tissue, and weight is gained. Weight is lost if caloric intake is reduced below the amount required for normal metabolic processes. It is sometimes said that obesity is due to a malfunction of the endocrine glands. In the vast majority of cases, obesity is the result of overeating and can be "cured" by reduction in food intake. In rare instances, hypothyroidism contributes to obesity because of reduction in the body's metabolic rate. Cushing's disease due to adrenal cortical hyperfunction may be associated with increased deposition of fat and an abnormal distribution of body fat. These are uncommon situations; almost all obese individuals have no detectable endocrine or metabolic disturbances.

COMPLICATIONS OF OBESITY

Overweight persons have a higher incidence of cardiovascular disease and many other diseases than persons of normal weight. Therefore, any degree of overweight is undesirable. Extreme obesity is a major health hazard; obese persons have a mortality rate almost twice that of normal individuals, for several reasons. The extremely obese individual requires a greatly increased blood volume and cardiac output to nourish the large mass of adipose tissue which serves no useful purpose. This is often associated with cardiac hypertrophy and may lead to congestive heart failure. Blood lipids are also frequently elevated in obese persons, one factor which predisposes them to premature atherosclerosis (Chapter 15).

Large masses of adipose tissue may impair normal pulmonary ventilation, producing various types of respiratory difficulty and increased susceptibility to pulmonary infection. An otherwise relatively minor illness may, in an obese person, be a catastrophe because of the increased demands placed upon already-overtaxed cardiovascular and respiratory systems.

When an obese person requires a surgical operation, the operative procedure carries a higher risk and postoperative complications are more frequent. Any surgical procedure is technically much more difficult in an obese person, and wound-healing is delayed. The adipose tissue, which has a relatively poor blood supply, heals poorly and is also quite vulnerable to infection, resulting in an increased incidence of postoperative wound infections.

Chapter 29

The Nervous System

THE CENTRAL NERVOUS SYSTEM consists of the brain and spinal cord, surrounded by several membranes called *meninges*. The brain is divided into the cerebrum, brain stem, and cerebellum. The brain is hollow, containing four interconnected cavities called *ventricles*. Arterial blood is supplied to the brain by large blood vessels entering the base of the skull. These arteries join to form a circle of vessels at the base of the brain, and branches from the circle extend outward to supply all parts of the brain. Venous blood is returned from the brain into large venous sinuses in the meninges, which eventually drain into the jugular veins. The brain and cord are surrounded by cerebrospinal fluid and are encased within protective bony structures, the cranium and vertebral column. The bony case protects the soft and rather fragile nervous tissue, and the cerebrospinal fluid acts as a hydrostatic cushion to insulate the brain from shocks and blows.

The brain and cord are composed of masses of nerve cells and nerve fibers. Each individual nerve cell has a central body and one or more long processes called *axons*, concerned with the transmission of the nerve impulses. Most nerve fibers are covered by a fatty insulating *myelin sheath*. A nerve which transmits impulses into the nervous system is called a *sensory nerve*. A *motor nerve* transmits impulses from brain or spinal cord to muscle. The *gray matter* of the brain and cord is composed primarily of masses of *nerve cell bodies;* the white matter consists mostly of *nerve fibers* covered by fatty myelin sheaths.

The nervous system may be considered as a giant switchboard, receiving sensory impulses and relaying this information to brain and spinal cord centers concerned with perception of sensation and with motor activity. The cerebral hemispheres control voluntary motor activity.

Normal muscles are never completely relaxed. Sensory impulses are being continually delivered to the central nervous system from nerve endings in muscles, joints, and tendons. Some impulses are conveyed to

173

cortical centers. Others establish connection with motor nerve cells within the spinal cord (often called "lower motor neurons") and cause discharge of motor impulses to the muscles. As a result of this reflex arc involving sensory input and lower motor neuron output, all muscles are in a continuous state of slight contractility called *muscle tone*. Voluntary motor activity in muscle is controlled by nerve impulses originating in motor neurons in the cerebral cortex (often called "upper motor neurons"). The nerve impulses descend in fiber tracts, establish contact with lower motor neurons in the cord, and induce discharge of motor impulses by the lower motor neurons, thereby initiating contraction of the voluntary muscle supplied by the motor nerve. Thus, muscle tone requires sensory input and an intact lower motor neuron cell and fiber. Voluntary motor activity requires participation of both cortical and spinal motor neurons.

Muscle Paralysis

A muscle which is no longer subject to voluntary control is said to be paralyzed. Two different types of paralysis are recognized: (1) *flaccid paralysis*, due to disease of the lower motor neuron or its nerve fiber, and (2) *spastic paralysis*, due to disease involving the cortical motor neurons or nerve fibers.

If the motor nerve cells in the spinal cord are destroyed by a disease, such as poliomyelitis, or if the peripheral nerve supplying the muscle (which represents the fibers of the spinal neurons) is damaged or interrupted, motor impulses to the muscles supplied by the affected nerves are interrupted, muscle tone is abolished, and the muscle rapidly undergoes marked atrophy. This is called *flaccid paralysis*.

If cortical motor nerve cells, or cortical nerve fibers passing downward to the cord, are injured within the brain, voluntary control of muscles supplied by the involved nerves and fibers is interrupted. However, the reflex arc concerned with muscle tone is not disturbed, and therefore muscle tone is not abolished. Marked atrophy of muscle does not develop. Usually tone is increased, since cortical impulses normally tend to inhibit muscle tone. This is called *spastic paralysis*.

Many neurologic diseases cause damage to cortical neurons or fiber tracts within the brain. Therefore, spastic paralysis is encountered more frequently than flaccid paralysis in medical practice.

Cerebral Injury

The brain is well protected from moderate trauma. However, it may be injured by a severe blow, and sometimes the skull is also fractured. Injury to the brain may be manifested by loss of consciousness and various neurologic disturbances. The injured brain becomes swollen and often shows evidence of pinpoint hemorrhages due to disruption of small intracerebral blood vessels. Usually the brain injury is located immediately adjacent to the site of the blow. However, sometimes the brain injury is due to violent contact of the displaced brain against the cranial cavity on the side opposite the injury. For example, the force of a blow to the back of the head may displace the brain forward within the cranial cavity, injuring the front of the brain where it strikes against the front of the bony cranial cavity.

Sometimes large blood vessels over the surface of the brain are torn by the force of the injury, and blood accumulates between the skull and the underlying brain. The expanding collection of blood, called a *hematoma,* may severely compress the underlying brain tissue.

Unfortunately, the rigid cranial cavity, which normally serves a protective function, is a disadvantage if the brain is seriously injured. This is because of the swelling of the brain which often occurs at the site of injury. The unyielding cranial cavity restricts the swelling, compresses the swollen brain, and leads to increased intracranial pressure. The elevated pressure adversely affects cerebral function and may also interfere with the blood supply to the brain by compressing cerebral blood vessels.

Stroke

The term *stroke* is used to designate any injury to brain tissue resulting from disturbance of blood supply to the brain. It may result from thrombosis of a cerebral artery due to arteriosclerosis or from rupture of an arteriosclerotic vessel and consequent cerebral hemorrhage. Rarely, a stroke is due to blockage of a cerebral artery by an embolus.

In cerebral thrombosis, which is more common than cerebral hemorrhage, the brain tissue in the area of distribution of the blocked vessel becomes necrotic and degenerates. The myelin sheath material undergoes breakdown, and the debris resulting from necrosis of brain tissue is eventually cleaned up by phagocytes, leaving a cystic cavity. Since the end stage of an infarct of brain is cystic, in contrast to the appearance of infarcts in other tissues, the term *encephalomalacia* (*encephalon* = brain + *malacia* = softening) is often used to refer to this type of lesion. Persons with high blood pressure are more susceptible to cerebral hemorrhage. Blood from the ruptured vessel escapes into the brain under high pressure and causes extensive damage to brain tissue. A large cerebral hemorrhage is frequently fatal.

A stroke is occasionally caused by an arteriosclerotic obstruction of one of the major arteries arising from the aorta, before the vessel enters the cranial cavity. Obstruction of the carotid artery in the neck is a common site of extracranial block. This markedly impairs cerebral blood flow and may cause a large cerebral infarction.

The clinical effects of a stroke depend primarily on the location of the brain damage and the amount of brain tissue injured. Frequently, the injury involves the large motor nerve fiber tracts descending from the cortex to the spinal cord. These fiber tracts cross in the brain stem, so that nerve cells from the right cerebral hemisphere supply the muscles on the left side of the body, and nerve cell bodies in the left side of the brain supply the muscles on the right side of the body. As a consequence, a brain injury is frequently manifested by a paralysis on the opposite side of the body.

Cerebral blood flow can be studied in the patient suspected of having cerebral or extracranial vascular disease by injection of a radiopaque dye into the arteries supplying the brain. The course of the dye is followed by serial x-ray studies, using the same type of methods applied to visualize the coronary arteries. Arteriosclerotic plaques which occlude the carotid artery and impede cerebral blood flow can be removed surgically.

Subarachnoid Hemorrhage

Subarachnoid hemorrhage refers to bleeding within the meninges. It is usually caused by rupture of a *congenital aneurysm* of one of the arteries making up the circle of vessels at the base of the brain. This has been discussed in the section on the cardiovascular system (Chapter 15).

Meningitis

Meningitis refers to an inflammation of the meninges surrounding the brain and spinal cord. Although a large number of organisms are capable of causing meningitis, most cases are due to infection caused by the *meningococcus, Hemophilus influenzae,* or the *pneumococcus.* The symptoms are those of a systemic infection, consisting of fever and increased numbers of leukocytes in the blood. In addition, there are signs of irritation of the central nervous system and of increased intracranial pressure: stiff neck, headache, sometimes convulsions, and coma. Diagnosis is established by examination of the spinal fluid, which contains large numbers of neutrophilic leukocytes and bacteria. Treatment consists of administration of appropriate antibiotics.

Hydrocephalus

Cerebrospinal fluid serves as a protective cushion around the brain and spinal cord. The fluid is secreted by the choroid plexuses of the lateral ventricles, passes into the third ventricle, through the cerebral aqueduct (aqueduct of Sylvius) into the fourth ventricle, and out of the ventricle through three small openings in the roof of the fourth ventricle. The fluid circulates around the cord and over the convexity of the brain and is re-absorbed into the large venous sinuses in the meninges. Obstruction to the normal circulation of spinal fluid distends the ventricles proximal to the site of the obstruction, with associated compression atrophy of brain tissue around the dilated ventricles. Hydrocephalus may be either congenital or acquired.

Congenital hydrocephalus is due to a congenital abnormality in the ventricular system, usually a congenital obstruction or abnormal formation of the cerebral aqueduct. This leads to marked distention of the lateral ventricles and third ventricle. Since the distention develops before the skull bones have fused, the head enlarges markedly, and the brain undergoes pronounced atrophy secondary to compression by the dilated ventricles.

Acquired hydrocephalus is most commonly caused by obstruction of the circulation of cerebrospinal fluid by postinflammatory fibrous adhesions in the region of the fourth ventricle, blocking the outflow of fluid from the fourth ventricle, or by blockage of the ventricular system secondary to a brain tumor. Acquired hydrocephalus develops after the fusion of the skull bones, so that the skull is incapable of enlargement, as in the congenital form of hydrocephalus.

Sometimes hydrocephalus can be treated by insertion of a plastic tube into the distended ventricle, the other end being placed beyond the site of obstruction.

Multiple Sclerosis

Multiple sclerosis is a chronic disease of unknown etiology characterized by the development of focal areas of degeneration of myelin sheaths of the nerve fibers in the brain and spinal cord. The lesions develop in a random manner throughout the brain and spinal cord. The areas of demyelination eventually heal by the formation of masses of glial scar tissue. The name of the disease is derived from the characteristic *multiple* areas of involvement which heal by *sclerosis* (another name for scarring). The glial scarring in this disease is produced by a type of neuroglial cell called an *astrocyte,* and differs somewhat from the usual fibrous scar produced by connective tissue cells.

Clinically, the disease is characterized by periodic episodes of acute neurological disturbances, the nature depending on the location of demyelination; this is followed by recovery and periods of remission. Eventually permanent neurologic disabilities occur as a consequence of the multiple areas of glial scarring, which impair conduction of nerve impulses in the brain and spinal cord.

Parkinson's Disease

Parkinson's disease is a chronic, disabling disease, characterized by rigidity of voluntary muscles and tremor of fingers and extremities. A number of drugs have been used successfully to control the symptoms of the disease.

Brain Tumors

Occasionally, a metastatic tumor may develop in the brain secondary to a primary malignant tumor in the breast, colon, lung, or other site. Primary brain tumors are relatively uncommon but may develop from the meninges, from the glial supporting tissues of the brain, or rarely from other tissues, such as blood vessels within the brain. A tumor of the meninges is called a *meningioma.* Any tumor of neuroglial origin is called a *glioma.* These tumors are further classified according to the type of glial supporting cell from which the neoplasm originated. Primary brain tumors do not metastasize, but many of the glial tumors carry with them a very poor prognosis because they often develop deep within the brain and are difficult to remove completely. The glial tumors are also quite resistant to radiation therapy.

The symptoms of a brain tumor depend on the size and location of the tumor. The patient may complain of a headache due to the increased intracranial pressure attending the increased volume of the intracranial contents. Or, any of various neurologic disturbances may manifest themselves due to disruption of nerve cells and fibers within the brain, secondary to the growth of the tumor.

Chapter 30

Skeletal and Articular System

THE SKELETON is the rigid supporting structure of the body. The bones are hollow, a method of construction providing a high degree of strength without excessive weight. Growth in length of bone takes place at the ends (epiphyses) of the bone. Increase in thickness is due to formation of new bone from the surrounding periosteum. In general, the strength and thickness of the bones depends on the activities of the individual. A man accustomed to strenuous physical labor has thicker, heavier bones than one who normally is engaged in light, sedentary activities. If an extremity is immobilized and is not allowed to bear weight, as after a fracture, the immobilized bones undergo marked thinning and decalcification, called *disuse atrophy.*

The bones of the skeleton are connected by means of joints. In a movable joint, the ends of the bones are covered with smooth articular cartilage and are held together by a fibrous joint capsule, reinforced by dense fibrous bands (ligaments). The joint capsule is lined by a thin syno-

Fig. 30-1.—Structure of a typical movable joint.

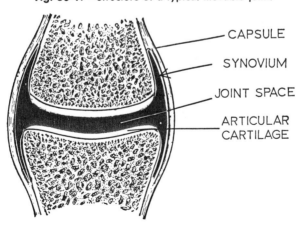

CAPSULE

SYNOVIUM

JOINT SPACE

ARTICULAR
CARTILAGE

TABLE 30-1.—COMPARISON OF MAJOR FEATURES OF COMMON TYPES
OF ARTHRITIS

	RHEUMATOID ARTHRITIS	OSTEOARTHRITIS	GOUT
Age and sex of patients most commonly affected	Young and middle-aged women	Elderly adults	Middle-aged men
Major characteristic of disease	A systemic disease with major effects in joints; causes chronic synovitis	"Wear-and-tear" degeneration of articular cartilage	Disturbance of nucleic acid metabolism; acute episodes due to crystals of uric acid in joints
Secondary effects of disease	Ingrowth of inflammatory tissue over cartilage destroys cartilage and leads to destruction of joint space; deformities common	Overgrowth of bone; thickening of periarticular soft tissues	Deposits of uric acid in joints with damage to joints (gouty arthritis); soft tissue tophi
Joints usually involved	Small joints of hands and feet	Major weight-bearing joints	Small joints; joint at base of great toe often involved
Special features	Autoantibody against gamma globulin (rheumatoid factor)	No systemic symptoms or biochemical abnormalities	High blood level of uric acid

vial membrane (the synovium), which secretes a small amount of mucinous fluid to lubricate the joint. Figure 30-1 illustrates the structure of a typical movable joint. In joint disease, these structures become altered as a result of inflammation or degeneration, leading to derangement in the functions of the joints.

Arthritis

Arthritis is one of the most common and disabling diseases of the skeletal system. Although there are many different kinds of arthritis, the three most common are *rheumatoid arthritis, osteoarthritis,* and *gout* (Table 30-1.)

RHEUMATOID ARTHRITIS

Rheumatoid arthritis is actually a systemic disease involving the connective tissues throughout the body, but the most pronounced clinical manifestations are in the joints. Clinically, the disease is seen as a chronic, disabling, and often deforming arthritis affecting multiple joints. The disease is encountered most frequently in young and middle-aged women; it usually involves the small joints of the hands and feet. In the joints, the disease produces a chronic inflammation and thickening of the synovial membrane. The inflammatory tissue extends over the surface of the articular cartilage, causing destruction of the joint cartilage. The marked damage to the articular surfaces makes the joint unstable; this in turn, leads to deviation or displacement of the bones due to the pull of the surrounding ligaments and tendons. Often fibrous adhesions develop within the joint, and the ends of the adjacent bones may become completely fused together. The end result of these various structural derangements is often severe disability and marked deformity of the affected joints.

The blood of patients with rheumatoid arthritis often contains a substance called *rheumatoid factor,* an autoantibody directed against one of the serum proteins (gamma globulin). It appears that this disease is related in some way to interaction between the autoantibody and the individual's own serum protein. Because of the systemic nature of this disease and the presence of autoantibodies, rheumatoid arthritis is often classified as one of the autoimmune diseases (Chapter 4).

The disease tends to fluctuate in severity. Periods of activity may alternate with intervals when the disease is inactive. Although there is no cure for rheumatoid arthritis, a number of measures are available which can control the disease and minimize its attending disability and deformity.

OSTEOARTHRITIS

In contrast to rheumatoid arthritis (a systemic disease), osteoarthritis represents "wear-and-tear" degeneration of one or more of the major weight-bearing joints. The disease is seen in older adults and may be considered as a manifestation of the normal aging process. The primary change in osteoarthritis is degeneration of the articular cartilage, leading to roughening of the articular surfaces of the bones. As a consequence, the bones grate against one another on motion of the joint, rather than gliding smoothly. Sometimes degeneration of the cartilage leaves large areas of underlying bone exposed. There is frequently secondary overgrowth of bone in response to the trauma of weight-bearing, and some thickening of the synovium and adjacent soft tissues also tends to occur. Clinically, persons with osteoarthritis experience stiffness, creaking, and some pain on motion of the joints. However, disability is not marked, and destruction of the joints does not occur.

Gout

Gout is a disorder of nucleic acid metabolism, seen most commonly in middle-aged men. The disease is characterized by excessive accumulation of uric acid in the body (an end product of nucleic acid breakdown). Usually the level of uric acid in the blood is also elevated. Clinically, the person afflicted with gout experiences periodic episodes of extremely painful arthritis involving a single joint, often the joint at the base of the great toe. The acute episodes are due to crystallization of uric acid within the joint; the crystals incite an acute inflammatory reaction. In untreated patients, eventually masses of uric acid crystals become deposited in and around the articular surfaces of the joints, injuring the joint surfaces; this is called *gouty arthritis*. Large, lumpy masses of uric acid crystals, called *gouty tophi*, are often deposited in the soft tissues around the joints and in other locations. Uric acid stones may form within the kidney and lower urinary tract due to crystallization of uric acid in the urine.

Treatment of gout consists of administering drugs which lower uric acid either by interfering with the formation of uric acid within the body or by promoting the excretion of uric acid by the kidneys. Acute attacks of gout can often be prevented by avoiding certain foods rich in nucleoprotein which tend to raise blood uric acid levels.

Table 30-1 compares the major features of these three types of arthritis.

Osteomyelitis

Acute inflammation of bone is called *osteomyelitis*. In children, bacteria may occasionally be carried in the bloodstream and lodge at the growing epiphyseal ends of bone, causing an acute inflammation. Osteomyelitis may also follow a compound fracture in which bacteria gain access to the fracture site through a laceration in the overlying skin.

Fracture

A fracture is a broken bone. In a *simple fracture,* the bone is broken in only two pieces. The term *comminuted fracture* is used when the bone is shattered into several pieces. A *compound fracture* is one in which the overlying skin has been broken. This is a more serious type of fracture because of the possibility of secondary bacterial invasion of the fracture site and development of osteomyelitis.

After a fracture, the ends of the broken bone may remain aligned, or they may be displaced out of position. The term "reduction of a fracture" refers to realigning the ends of the broken bone so that the bone will heal in its normal anatomic position. Sometimes this can be accomplished by means of manipulation of the injured extremity to realign the ends of the bone, after which the extremity is immobilized in a plaster cast. However, sometimes a surgical operation must be performed to reduce the fracture and hold it in position by means of a metal plate and screws, or similar device. This is called an "open reduction." Sometimes a bone may become so weakened by disease, such as metastatic tumor, that it breaks after minimal stress (for example, coughing or sneezing). A fracture of this type through a diseased area in bone is called a "pathologic fracture."

Bone Tumors

Bone is often involved by metastatic tumors. Carcinoma of breast or prostate, as well as many other tumors, frequently metastasize to bone. Occasionally, the skeletal system may be so heavily infiltrated by tumor that hematopoietic cells within the marrow are crowded out, leading to anemia, leukopenia, and thrombocytopenia (Chapter 16). Nodular deposits of neoplastic plasma cells are frequently present throughout the skeletal system in *multiple myeloma* (Chapter 12). Benign cysts and primary tumors of bone are encountered occasionally, but primary malignant tumors of bone are rare.

Osteoporosis

Osteoporosis, literally meaning "porous bones," is a generalized thinning and demineralization of the entire skeletal system. Most cases occur in postmenopausal women beginning in the fifth decade, and a significant degree of osteoporosis is said to be present in approximately one fourth of all women by the sixth decade. Because of the high incidence of the disease in postmenopausal women, it is thought that the decreased levels of estrogen following the menopause contribute in some way to the demineralization of bone. Osteoporosis also occurs in elderly men, but develops at a much later age and usually is less marked than in women.

The osteoporotic bones are quite fragile and susceptible to fracture. Fractures of vertebral bodies occur frequently, either due to the stress of weight-bearing or after minor exertion. This produces back pain and tenderness. Such fractures are often characterized by collapse of the anterior portions of the vertebral bodies (compression fractures). Collapse of vertebral bodies may compress the spinal nerve roots passing through the intervertebral foramina, leading to radiating pain along the course of the compressed nerve.

Treatment of osteoporosis consists of various measures to control pain and disability due to fractures, together with administration of a high calcium diet and other measures which promote increased deposition of bone.

Avascular Necrosis

Occasionally the growing cartilaginous ends of bone (epiphyses) in children and adolescents undergo necrosis and degeneration, due to interference with the blood supply to the epiphysis. This is termed *avascular necrosis*. Sometimes this follows an injury, but in most cases the reason for the vascular disturbance is unknown. Common sites of avascular necrosis are the femoral head, the tibial tubercle, the articular surface of the femoral condyle, and occasionally the small bones of the ankle and foot. Symptoms consist of pain and disability related to motion of the affected joint.

Disease of the Spinal Intervertebral Disks

The intervertebral disks are fibrocartilaginous cushions interposed between adjacent surfaces of the vertebral bodies (Fig. 30-2, left). An intervertebral disk is composed of a central mass of soft, extremely elastic tissue called the *nucleus pulposus* ("pulpy nucleus"), surrounded by a dense ring of fibrous tissue and cartilage termed the *annulus fibrosus* ("fibrous ring"). The intervertebral disks function as shock absorbers. Under pressure, the highly elastic nucleus pulposus becomes compressed and pushes outward against the more resistant annulus, absorbing the force of compression and preventing direct impact between adjacent vertebral bodies.

The intervertebral disks undergo a progressive wear-and-tear type of degenerative change with advancing age, involving both the nucleus pulposus and the annulus. The nucleus loses elasticity and becomes brittle; the annulus becomes weakened and thinned. The posterior part of the weakened annulus may rupture as a result of stress related to lifting or straining; this causes extrusion of portions of the degenerated nucleus pulposus into the spinal canal (Fig. 30-2, right). Generally, the protrusion of disk material occurs in the lumbosacral region. This is because the spinal curvature is greatest and the disks are subject to the most marked mechanical stresses in this area. Usually the disk material is extruded in a posterolateral direction, often impinging on lumbosacral nerve roots. Symptoms of disk protrusion (sometimes called a "slipped disk") consist of sudden onset of acute back pain after an episode of lifting or other exertion. Frequently, the pain is also felt in the leg and thigh, representing radiation of pain along the course of the nerve compressed by the protruded disk. Treatment consists of bed rest and various other measures to minimize pain

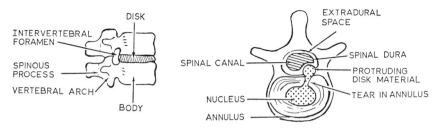

Fig. 30-2.—**Left,** relationship of intervertebral disks to vertebral bodies, interverte-bral foramina, and spinal canal. Spinal cord and spinal nerve roots lie within the spinal canal dorsal to the vertebral bodies, surrounded by the spinal dura, and pro-tected by the vertebral arches. Spinal nerve roots penetrate spinal dura and pass through the intervertebral foramina. **Right,** cross-section through the vertebral column at level of intervertebral disk, illustrating the usual anatomic relationships in a protru-sion of disk material. Portions of degenerated nucleus pulposus are extruded through a tear in the annulus fibrosus, impinging on the dural sac and nerve roots external to the dura.

and disability. Protruded disk material may undergo resorption, and the tear in the annulus is repaired by fibrous tissue. Sometimes surgical re-moval of the protruded disk material may be required.

It is usually possible to demonstrate the protrusion of the disk material into the spinal canal by means of a special radiologic procedure called a *myelogram.* Radiopaque material is introduced into the dural sac sur-rounding the cord and nerve roots, in order to outline the contour of the dural sac. The location of the disk material can be recognized in the x-ray film as a filling defect in the column of radiopaque material.

Chapter 31

Skeletal Muscle

MUSCLE CELLS are highly specialized contractile cells. Three different types of muscle are recognized: involuntary muscle, skeletal muscle, and cardiac muscle. Involuntary muscle is present in the walls of the gastrointestinal tract, biliary tract, urogenital system, respiratory tract, and blood vessels. Skeletal muscle is attached to the skeleton by means of tendons and ligaments; it is concerned with voluntary muscular activity. Cardiac muscle closely resembles skeletal muscle, but has certain special features related to its function of producing rhythmic contractions of the heart. Lesions of involuntary muscles are rare, and disorders of cardiac muscle have already been considered in Chapter 15. A discussion of skeletal muscle, the great bulk of muscle within the body, follows.

Contraction of Skeletal Muscle

The contractility of the muscle cell is due to the presence of long filaments called *myofibrils*, composed of specialized contractile protein. The fibrils fill the cytoplasm of the muscle cell and are arranged parallel to the long axis of the cell. The cytoplasm also contains a large number of energy-rich organic compounds, ions, and enzymes required for the metabolic activity of the muscle cell.

Muscle cells contract in response to motor nerve impulses conveyed to the muscle. The area of communication between the nerve endings and the muscle cell is called the *myoneural junction*. The actual stimulation of the muscle cell is due to a chemical called *acetylcholine* which is released from the nerve endings at the myoneural junction. The chemical mediator acetylcholine initiates the biochemical chain of events leading to shortening of the myofibrils, which, in turn, results in contraction of the muscle cell. The duration of action of the chemical mediator is quite brief because of the rapid breakdown of this substance by the enzyme *cholinesterase*, present in muscle and in the blood.

Factors Influencing Muscle Structure and Function

The normal structural and functional integrity of skeletal muscle depends on an intact nerve supply, normal transmission of impulses across the myoneural junction, and normal metabolic processes within the muscle cell.

As has been considered previously (Chapter 29), skeletal muscle is normally in a continuous state of slight contractility, called *muscle tone.* Muscles which are not used, or muscles deprived of their nerve supply, undergo marked atrophy. Conversely, muscles which perform increased work undergo hypertrophy in response to the increased demands.

Muscle cells contain a highly complex metabolic machinery capable of translating nerve impulses into muscle contractions. Any disturbance in the metabolism of the muscle cell leads to a disturbance in the function of the cell. The intracellular metabolic processes are also influenced by the various endocrine glands regulating the rate of metabolism within the muscle cell and influencing the concentration of the various ions required for normal muscle contraction.

Diseases of Skeletal Muscle

Diseases of skeletal muscle are uncommon. The main disorders consist of muscular atrophy, degeneration of muscle, disturbance of impulse conduction at the myoneural junction, and inflammatory lesions.

INFLAMMATION OF MUSCLE (MYOSITIS)

LOCALIZED MYOSITIS.—Small areas of inflammation in skeletal muscle are encountered in a large number of systemic diseases and have no major clinical significance. Inflammation of muscle may also follow injury or muscular overexertion. The inflammation is secondary to necrosis and disruption of muscle cells and is associated with swelling and tenderness of the affected muscle. The inflammation gradually subsides as the muscle injury heals.

GENERALIZED MYOSITIS.—Generalized inflammation of skeletal muscle (*polymyositis*) is an uncommon but serious systemic disease of unknown etiology, characterized by widespread degeneration and inflammation of skeletal muscle. One type of polymyositis, associated with swelling and inflammation of the skin, is called *dermatomyositis.* These disorders are often classified as collagen diseases (Chapter 4) because of the necrosis of connective tissue fibers in the involved muscles, and because these diseases are presumed to have an immunologic basis.

HEREDITARY DISEASES CHARACTERIZED BY ATROPHY
AND DEGENERATION OF MUSCLE

Several relatively rare hereditary diseases are characterized by progressive atrophy or degeneration of skeletal muscles. Various clinical syndromes are recognized, depending on the muscle groups involved, the patterns of inheritance, and the rate of progression of the disease. In general, these diseases are characterized by marked muscle weakness and progressive atrophy of skeletal muscles, resulting in gradually increasing disability and eventually terminating in death due to paralysis of the respiratory muscles or superimposed respiratory infection. The hereditary diseases fall into two large groups. In one group, called *progressive muscular atrophy*, the muscular weakness and atrophy are due to progressive degeneration of nerve cells in the cerebral cortex, brain stem, and spinal cord. In the second group, the nerve supply to the muscle is unaffected. The basic disturbance lies in the metabolic processes within the muscle cells, leading to actual necrosis and degeneration of individual muscle cells. These latter diseases are grouped under the term *muscular dystrophy*. In the most common type of muscular dystrophy, the disease becomes manifest during early childhood and usually progresses relatively rapidly, resulting in death during adolescence or early adulthood. The muscles primarily involved are those concerned with motion of the trunk, lower extremities, hips, and shoulder girdle. Often the extent of atrophy is masked because of replacement of the atrophic muscles by fat, and the extent of fat infiltration may at times be so marked that the affected muscles appear hypertrophied. This leads to the paradox of an individual with profound muscular weakness whose muscles appear very well developed. The apparent hypertrophy is an illusion due to infiltration of the muscles by fat.

While the various types of muscular atrophy and muscular dystrophy are uncommon, they are of major concern not only to the patient, but to the family, because of the hereditary nature of many of these illnesses. There is no way at present to arrest the relentless progression of these diseases, but a number of measures can be taken to minimize the disability and prolong the life of affected individuals.

MYASTHENIA GRAVIS

Myasthenia gravis is a chronic disease characterized by abnormal fatigability of voluntary muscles. Fatigue develops rapidly when the muscles are used and subsides when they are rested. Often the dysfunction is most conspicuous in the small muscles of the face and in the muscles concerned with eye movement (extraocular muscles). The symptoms of the disease appear to be related to impaired transmission of impulses across the myoneural junction; they can be relieved by drugs which inhibit the action of the enzyme cholinesterase, thereby potentiating the action of the chemical mediator acetylcholine. Many patients with myasthenia gravis have been found to have either a tumor or a benign hyperplasia of the thymus gland. However, the exact relationship of the myasthenia to the abnormality of the thymus gland has not been elucidated. Removal of the thymus gland often has little effect on the disease.

Selected References for Further Study

BELOW is a brief list of reference books which the student will find useful for further study after a basic knowledge of the subject has been acquired. The list of references is not exhaustive. A recommended "core" reference library for persons in the health sciences has been published (Stearn, N. S., *et al.*: New England J. Med. 283:1489, 1970) and should be consulted if a more comprehensive listing of reference texts is required.

Pathology
Ackerman, L. V., and Del Regato, J. A.: *Cancer: Diagnosis, Treatment, and Prognosis* (4th ed.; St. Louis: C. V. Mosby Co., 1968).
Anderson, W. A. D.: *Pathology* (5th ed.; St. Louis: C. V. Mosby Co., 1966).
Boyd, W.: *Textbook of Pathology* (8th ed.; Philadelphia: Lea & Febiger, 1969).
Novak, E. R., and Woodruff, J. D.: *Novak's Gynecologic and Obstetric Pathology* (6th ed.; Philadelphia: W. B. Saunders Co., 1967).
Potter, E. L.: *Pathology of the Fetus and Infant* (2nd ed.; Chicago: Year Book Medical Publishers, 1961).
Robbins, S. L.: *Pathology* (3rd ed.; Philadelphia: W. B. Saunders Co., 1967).

Medicine
Beeson, P. B., and McDermott, W.: *Cecil-Loeb Textbook of Medicine* (13th ed.; Philadelphia: W. B. Saunders Co., 1971).
Conant, N., *et al.*: *Manual of Clinical Mycology* (2nd ed.; Philadelphia: W. B. Saunders, 1954).
Davenport, H. W.: *ABC of Acid-Base Chemistry* (5th ed.; Chicago: University of Chicago Press, 1969).
Harrison, T. R., *et al.*: *Principles of Internal Medicine* (6th ed.; New York: McGraw-Hill Book Co., 1970).

Hematology, Blood Groups, Hemolytic Disease
Charles, A. G., and Friedman, E. A.: *Rh Isoimmunization and Erythroblastosis Fetalis* (New York: Appleton-Century-Crofts, Inc., 1969).
Leavell, B. S., and Thorup, O. A.: *Fundamentals of Clinical Hematology* (2nd ed.; Philadelphia: W. B. Saunders Co., 1966).

Mollison, P. L.: *Blood Transfusion in Clinical Medicine* (4th ed.; Philadelphia: Blackwell-Davis Co., 1967).

Ratnoff, O.: *Bleeding Syndromes* (Springfield, Ill.: Charles C Thomas Co., 1960).

Genetics, Congenital Abnormalities

Carter, C. O.: *An ABC of Medical Genetics* (Boston: Little, Brown & Co., 1970).

McKusick, V.: *Human Genetics* (2nd ed.; Englewood Cliffs, N. J.: Prentice-Hall, Inc., 1969).

Physiology, Biochemistry, Pathologic Physiology, Endocrine Physiology

Best, C. H., and Taylor, N. B.: *The Living Body* (New York: Holt Rinehart & Winston, 1958).

Karlson, P.: *Introduction to Modern Biochemistry* (3rd ed.; New York: Academic Press, Inc., 1968).

Sawin, C. T.: *Hormones: Endocrine Physiology* (Boston: Little, Brown & Co., 1969).

Sodeman, W. A.: *Pathologic Physiology* (4th ed.; Philadelphia: W. B. Saunders Co., 1967).

Tepperman, J.: *Metabolic and Endocrine Physiology* (2nd ed.; Chicago: Year Book Medical Publishers, 1968).

Index

193

growth, 161
pituitary, secretion
abnormalities of, 163
physiologic control of, 162
thyroid
actions of, 163-164
goiter and, 165-167
-stimulating (TSH), 161
Host, 6
Humoral defense reaction, 9-10
Hydatidiform mole, 113
Hydrocephalus, 177
acquired, 177
congenital, 177
Hydrocortisone, 167
Hydronephrosis, 125
Hydrops fetalis, 114
Hydrostatic pressure: increased, and edema, 66
Hydrothorax, 65, 124
Hydroureter, 125
Hydroxylases, 169
Hyperplasia
adrenal, congenital, 169
endometrial, 110
prostatic, benign, 129
Hypersensitivity, 8-11
antibiotics and, 25
tuberculin-type, 11
Hypertension, 76-77
cardiac effects, 76-77
cause of, 77
portal, 137
renal effects, 77
treatment of, 77
vascular effects, 77
Hypertensive cardiovascular disease, 76-77
Hyperthyroidism, 164-165
comparison to hypothyroidism, 164
Hyperventilation, 158
Hypothyroidism, 165
comparison to hyperthyroidism, 164

I

Immune
autoimmune (see Autoimmune)
defense mechanism, cell-mediated, 10
reactions and lymphatic system, 94
Immunity, 8-11
acquired, 8
lymphocyte and, 8-9
mechanism of production of, 9
cell-mediated, 8
humoral immunity and, 9

grafts and, tissue, 11
humoral, 8
cell-mediated immunity and, 9
Immunization, 38
Immunologic defenses: against neoplasms, 56-57
Inclusion bodies: of virus disease, 30
Infarction, 62
myocardial, treatment of, 73-74
Infection
bacterial, and antibiotics (see Antibiotics)
chronic, 6-7
definition of, 4-5
fungal, 27-28
maternal, 45
outcome of, factors influencing, 6
tuberculous, course of, 100, 101
viral (see Virus(es), infection)
Infectious hepatitis, 134
Infectious mononucleosis, 93-94
Inflammation, 4-7
granulomatous, 100
lymph nodes, 92
muscle (see Myositis)
Inflammatory
disease, 2
intestinal, 146-147
process, 4-5
reaction, definition, 4
Injury
cerebral, 174-175
to liver, 133-134
causes of, 133
effects of, 133
necrosis due to (see Necrosis, cell, injury causing)
renal tubular, 124-125
Insulin: and diabetes mellitus, 141
Intestine
inflammatory disease of, 146-147
obstruction, 148-149
causes of, 148-149
high, 148
low, 148
Intrinsic factor, 86
Iodine: deficiency, and goiter, 165
Iron: -deficiency anemia, 85-86
Islets of Langerhans, 140, 171
Isolation: and communicable disease, 38

J

Jaundice, 138-139
hemolytic, 139

Sodium bicarbonate (*see* Bicarbonate)
Spastic paralysis, 174
Spinal intervertebral disks: disease of, 184-185
Spiral organisms, 20-21
Staphylococci, 18
Stenosis, 71
Sterol, 75
Stomach: carcinoma of, 146
Stomatitis, 144
Streptococci, 18
    gamma, 18
    hemolytic
        alpha, 18
        beta, 18
    nonhemolytic, 18
Stricture: esophageal, 145
Stroke, 175-176
Subarachnoid hemorrhage, 176
Symptoms: definition of, 1

T

Tapeworms, 35-36
Teratoma, 50
Testis: carcinoma of, 130
Tetanus, 19
Tetany, 171
Thorax
    hydrothorax, 65, 124
    pneumothorax, 98
    wall, relationship to lung, 98
Thrombocytopenia, 60, 86, 90-91
    primary, 91
    secondary, 91
Thromboplastic material: liberation into circulation, 61
Thromboplastin formation
    extrinsic system of, 59
    intrinsic system of, 59
Thrombosis, 62-65
    arterial, 63
    coagulation and, 64
    intracardiac, 63-64
    mesenteric, 149
    venous, 62-63
Thrombus: definition of, 62
Thyroid, 163-167
    function, abnormalities of, 164-165
    hormone (*see* Hormone, thyroid)
Thyroiditis, 167
    chronic, 167
Thyrotoxicosis, 164
Tissue: grafts and immunity, 11
Tophi: gouty, 182
Toxicity: antibiotic, 24-25

Transfusions and hemolytic disease (*see* Hemolytic disease, transfusions and)
Trauma (*see* Injury)
Treponema pallidum, 20, 25
Trichinella, 34, 35
    spiralis, 35
Triglyceride, 75
Trisomy, 41
Trisomy 21, 41
TSH (thyroid-stimulating hormone), 161
Tuberculin-type hypersensitivity, 11
Tuberculosis, 100-102
    diagnosis of, 102
    extrapulmonary, 101-102
    miliary, 101
    treatment of, 102
Tuberculous
    infection, course of, 100, 101
    pneumonia, 101
Tubule (*see* Kidney, tubule)
Tumors, 49-57
    adrenal sex-hormone-producing, 169
    benign, 48-49
        comparison to malignant, 49
    bone, 183
    brain, 178
    cytologic diagnosis of, 51-52
    early recognition of, 54-55
    embryonic, 50-51
    frozen section diagnosis of, 55
    gallbladder, 138
    hepatic, 138
    immunologic defenses against, 56-57
    lymph nodes and, 93
    lymphoid, 50
    malignant (*see* Cancer)
    of mixed components, 50
    ovarian, 110-111
    pancreatic, 140
    of pigment-producing epithelium, 50
    prostatic, 129-130
    terminology, 49-51
        general principles of, 49
        variations in, 50-51
    treatment of, 55
    urinary tract, 126
    viruses and, 55
    Wilms', 126

U

Ulcer; chronic peptic, 145-146
Uremia, 127
Urinary casts, 122